鄭子太極拳十三篇

The Annotated Thirteen Chapters

Master Cheng's
Thirteen Chapters
on T'ai-Chi Ch'üan

Published by
Sweet Ch'i Press
662 Union St.
Brooklyn, New York 11215

Copyright ©1982 by Douglas Wile
ISBN 0-912059-00-1

First Edition, summer, 1982.
Second printing (with corrections), fall, 1982.
Third printing (with revisions), spring, 1983.
Fourth printing, winter, 1984.

15   14   13   12   11   10   9   8   7

*For Chow Tse-tsung
who taught me the Way of scholarship.*

ACKNOWLEDGMENTS

Special thanks for this edition to
Marsha Bain, William Brown, Janet
Christie-Wile, Lee Ching-tse, Zack Rogow.

TABLE OF CONTENTS

Translator's Note to First Edition   ix

Translator's Note to Fifth Edition   xi

Biography of Man-jan   1

Author's Preface   5

Chapter 1:   The Meaning of "T'ai-chi"   7

Chapter 2:   Understanding the Mysterious and
              the Substantial   10

Chapter 3:   Concentrating the *Ch'i* and
              Developing Softness   16

Chapter 4:   Transforming One's Disposition   20

Chapter 5:   Swimming on Dry Land   22

Chapter 6:   The Equal Importance of Heart
              and Spine   27

Chapter 7:   Energy and Physics   31

Chapter 8:   Cultivating Life and Maintaining
              Purity   43

Chapter 9:   Strengthening the Internal Organs   46

Chapter 10:   Curing Tuberculosis   49

Chapter 11:   Defining the Stages of Development   60

Chapter 12:   Elucidating Production and
              Destruction   67

Chapter 13:   Exposition of the Oral Transmission   72

Notes   81

Index   99

TRANSLATOR'S NOTE
TO THE FIRST EDITION

Cheng Man-ch'ing's *Master Cheng's Thirteen Chapters on T'ai-chi ch'üan* (Cheng Tzu T'ai-chi ch'üan shih-san p'ien) was completed in 1946, exactly a decade after the death of his teacher, Yang Ch'eng-fu. In his Preface to the work Cheng tells us that Yang was extremely reluctant to commit his teachings to print. However, in 1925 Yang's student, Ch'en Wei-ming, published a book entitled *The Art of T'ai-chi ch'üan* (T'ai-chi ch'üan shu) based on Yang's oral instruction and with photographs of the master. This was followed in the early 30's with two books published in Yang's own name: *The Complete Theory and Practice of T'ai chi ch'üan* (T'ai-chi ch'üan t'i-yung ch'üan-shu) and *Self-Defense Methods of T'ai-chi ch'üan* (T'ai-chi ch'üan shih-yung fa). In Chapter 13 of the *Thirteen Chapters* Cheng confides that he too was torn between his desire to share the benefits of T'ai-chi ch'üan with the world and his fear of its secrets falling into the "wrong" hands. For both men, trepidations were finally overcome by their deep commitment to the role they hoped T'ai-chi ch'üan could play in China's struggle for national revival.

Unlike Yang Ch'eng-fu, Professor Cheng was a member of the literati and a man of many parts. Bringing to T'ai-chi ch'üan his background in art, philosophy, literature, Chinese medicine and Western science, the *Thirteen Chapters* is marked by the sweep and synthesis of Cheng's remarkable renaissance mind.

Cheng's books on T'ai-chi ch'üan in Chinese and English since the publication of the *Thirteen Chapters* have been mainly a response to difficulties encountered by students in understanding the earlier work. Thus his advanced teachings were published first, while later writings were progressively simpler and more accessible, although by 1946 he had already shortened and modified the form to what is generally known as the "short Yang form."

It is now nearly twenty years since Professor Cheng brought his art to the West. The seeds planted in New York have flowered and born new seeds which have taken wing and sprouted in every corner of the continent and around the world. This far flung empire still honors its ancestors; yet as the *I ching* says, "The flight of dragons is without a head." Decentralization of authority since Cheng's death has opened the field for what looks at one moment like Warring States chaos and at another like an opportunity for cross pollination and further development.

Yang Ch'eng-fu regretted having scoffed at T'ai-chi in his youth, realizing his folly only after his father's death, and Cheng lamented his failure to take full advantage of Yang's knowledge while the master was still alive. This translation of the *Thirteen Chapters* was undertaken in the hope that as we approach the tenth anniversary of the Professor's passing, the movement of all those who identify with his transmission will be even better able to appreciate and profit from the fullness of his contribution. Leaving out some introductory material, form explanations, and commentaries the translation contains only the core "thirteen chapters" themselves. May it give joy and sustenance to its readers and new impetus to the art.

Prof. Douglas Wile
Brooklyn College
Fall, 1982

TRANSLATOR'S NOTE
TO THE FIFTH EDITION

This new edition of the first English translation of Cheng Man-ch'ing's *Thirteen Chapters* coincides with the 20th anniversary of his "mission" to the West and the 10th anniversary of his passing. In his writings, Cheng spoke both as prophet and as cultural ambassador. Like a prophet he passionately recalled his countrymen to their finest traditions, and like a cultural ambassador he skillfully employed the arts of China to promote an appreciation of Chinese culture in the West. This two-pronged thrust is consistent with the Confucian commitment to preserving and transmitting the traditions of "high" culture and to extending its "civilizing" influence to the rest of the world. Thus the *Thirteen Chapters* provides not only a microscopic view of the art of T'ai-chi ch'üan itself, but a fish-eye panorama of the whole landscape of China's intellectual heritage. T'ai-chi is a wonderful window for exploring this territory—philosophy, art and science are all there—and what better guide-book than the *Thirteen Chapters*?

The breadth of Cheng's erudition and the scope of his achievements (calligraphy, painting, poetry, martial arts, and medicine) makes the *Thirteen Chapters* an exceptionally rich but formidable work. Cheng's teaching was the fruit of the great tree of Chinese culture. The notes appended to this edition of the *Thirteen Chapters* attempt to sketch in the many branches of learning which produced and sustained that fruit. However universal its principles, the *Thirteen Chapters* is not a work out of time. The accompanying notes can help provide historical perspective—a sense of the roots of the work and how it responded to the needs of the nation. Far from emerging in an historical vacuum, the *Thirteen Chapters* was written in 1946, a period of intense social and political upheaval: ten years of Japanese occupation, twenty years of civil war, and a hundred years of Western intervention in China's affairs. Indeed, Cheng's lifetime stretches from the last years of the Manchu dynasty to the Warlord Epoch, Republic, People's Republic, exile in Taiwan, and conquest of the New World. The exigencies of the age are reflected in significant but subtle ways in the work, easily overlooked without supporting annotations.

Born in 1900, five years before the abolition of the imperial examination system, Cheng's writing bristles with the influence of an early classical education. Interestingly, the tenor of his thought is closer to the visionary reformers of a generation earlier — men like K'ang Yu-wei, T'an Ssu-t'ung and Liang Ch'i-ch'ao who reinterpreted tradition in order to resuscitate it — rather than the radical iconoclasts of his own generation whose May Fourth Movement (1919) called for wholesale Westernization and destruction of every artifact of the "feudal" society. This reactionary-reformist tension is reflected in Cheng's writing style, archaic and unreconciled with the vernacular literature movement, even while absorbing Western terminology and innovating within the native tradition. This nuance of language expresses an important aspect of Cheng's character and philosophical stance and calls for sensitive treatment in the style and diction of the translation.

The format of this revised *Thirteen Chapters* with annotations and index answers a number of specific purposes. First, since the publication of our earlier editions and subsequent translations of Yang family and additional Cheng material, it has become apparent that an increasingly sophisticated readership demands primary sources presented in a manner consistent with the standards of modern scholarship. Drawing as it does upon the author's deep knowledge of history, philosophy, meditation, medicine, and T'ai-chi ch'üan itself, the *Thirteen Chapters* is a challenging work for even native Chinese readers. For Westerners, notes are indispensable if much of the work's specialized terminology, quotes and allusions are not to be lost in obscurity. Secondly, translation is intrinsically an act of interpretation. If standards of translation for T'ai-chi texts are to be raised to a par with other disciplines, then the critical choices which every translator makes for the reader must be shared with and justified to the reader. This is a contribution translation can make not only to the readership, but to the dignity of T'ai-chi ch'üan itself. A third purpose envisioned for this annotated edition of the *Thirteen Chapters* is to help retrace the footsteps of the author's thought and to expose the matrix of his mind. Without glimpsing the process of Cheng's creation and the complex synthesis of sciences which produced it, can we hope to comprehend the work, much less be worthy successors?

Cheng drew on a number of distinct language provinces in the writing of the *Thirteen Chapters*. First are the literary and historical allusions which formed the stock in trade of the Chinese literati for perhaps three thousand years. Some of these are clearly introduced as quotes in the text, but most are simply the unconscious idiom of the educated elite. These are chiefly references to historical figures and expressions or passages from the Confucian and Taoist classics. A large number have been identified and noted in this new edition, both to illuminate the sources of Cheng's thought and to stimulate interest in further study of Chinese history and philosophy. The "T'ai-chi Classics" and special terminology of the martial arts are another language province drawn upon. Cheng again weaves these into his own text, either as citations or simply in passing, revealing both the utmost reverence for this slim corpus of canonical works and the degree of their assimilation into his own thinking. These quotes have been set off and the sources noted in order to allow interested readers to refer to the original context for clarification. A third language province Cheng tapped in the writing of his *Thirteen Chapters* is the metaphysical jargon derived from the *I ching* and developed by later commentators and philosophers such as Chou Tun-i and Shao Yung. *T'ai-chi, yin/yang,* the trigrams, hexagrams and Five Phases are to Chinese science what mathematics is to Western science, and Cheng makes extensive use of these to express relationships in the martial as well as meditational aspects of T'ai-chi ch'üan. Another specialized vocabulary often requiring explanatory notes belongs to China's sub-culture of Taoist self-cultivators. This is the most arcane of the language provinces and leans heavily on the symbolism of myth, alchemy, and the *I ching* to express super-normal psychic states and the movement and transformation of energy within the body. Equally inaccessible without detailed annotation is the language of traditional Chinese medicine. Cheng, himself a noted physician, was able to integrate medicine and martial art with a degree of insight and originality which redefined the very content of T'ai-chi ch'üan. A final language province is Western science, chiefly medicine and physics, which Cheng used ambivalently both to buttress his own assertions and to disparage in comparison with China's older sciences.

Writings on T'ai-chi ch'üan have evolved a number of distinct genres over the indeterminate period of its existence. It is possible to distinguish at least three major phases of the development of this literature, a progression which parallels the shift from private to public dissemination of texts. As with other Chinese arts, e.g., poetry, painting, or calligraphy, antecedent forms are retained cumulatively while newer modes of presentation simply expand the repertoire. China's literature of the arts of self-cultivation, however difficult to classify in traditional Western terms, nevertheless reveals some of the most subtle and powerful use of language ever conceived. The first genre phase of T'ai-chi "literature," then, if you will, includes posture sequences (*p'u*), classics (*ching*), treatises (*lun*), mnemonic verses (*chüeh*), and training songs (*ko*). These are characterized by high density, verse forms of varying meters, or rhythmic parallel prose. Many are difficult to date, sometimes anonymous, or variously attributed to different masters in different sources. It is safer to say that most existed as oral transmissions or holographs before appearing in print. The next phase includes commentaries to the classics by later masters or efforts by disciples to systematically record the principles and training methods of their teachers. The last genre to emerge consists of new martial forms synthesized from several schools or creative extension of one line of transmission presented in literary or modern expository style. All three genres have used graphic illustration and later photography in addition to written text.

The complete *Thirteen Chapters* contains elements of all three phases of the development of T'ai-chi literature. Cheng reproduced the Yang family recension of the "classics" and also included transcriptions of some of Yang Ch'eng-fu's oral instructions along with his own commentary. The body of the core "thirteen chapters" contains countless quotes from the T'ai-chi Classics, while the "Questions and Answers" section of the complete work is essentially a selected commentary to the "classics" in the form of a dialogue with students. What makes Cheng's *Thirteen Chapters* unique is that it goes beyond predictable metaphysical clichés and mere mechanical description of a martial form to a detailed exposition of traditional principles and teaching techniques together with his own highly original set of new conceptual tools for working in the medium of movement. Only a direct connection with the well-spring was capable of producing such fresh water. The published writings of such representative contemporaries as Sun Lu-t'ang (1919), Hsü Yü-sheng (1921), Ch'en Wei-ming (1925), Wu T'u-nan (1925) or Sung Shih-yüan (1946) appear by comparison colorless and one-dimensional. Cheng's use of medicine, meditation, Western science, and the patriotic imperative is also far more extensive and penetrating.

Cheng Man-ch'ing's *Thirteen Chapters* is a complex and multi-leveled work. In very orthodox terms, he strove to align T'ai-chi ch'üan with the broad Confucian and early Taoist enterprise of sagehood and rulership, to reunite the civil and the martial, and once and for all remove its lower class stigma. Going further, he held out the possibility of realizing the later Taoist esoteric goal of immortality through the techniques of inner alchemy. He was also uniquely qualified to develop the theoretical and practical application of T'ai-chi ch'üan in preventive and therapeutic medicine. Through his teaching and writings, he helped establish T'ai-chi ch'üan as part of the popular program of national self-strengthening and as a model of successful military strategy. Finally, he sought to demonstrate the superiority of traditional Chinese arts over Western techniques both to hearten his countrymen and later to educate the West.

This much is susceptible to analysis, but we must never overlook the genius of the man, his profound grasp of the art, and his ability to communicate its principles in relevant language. Cheng's contribution goes beyond his writings, beyond his pioneering mission to America, the number of teachers he trained, his much imitated concept of a simplified form, or even the subtle stylistic changes he introduced in the form, but goes to the essence of the art itself. His changes were not a case of "painting legs on snakes," but a truer image of the snake. The T'ai-chi teacher's function is to point towards the *tao*. The mature student does not cling to the pointing finger, but follows it like the needle of a compass. As a model, the teacher may be compared to the carpenter's square which is static, subjective, and only as good as its manufacture. The level and plumb, however, always refer directly to nature. The level is located in the head and the plumb line in the spine. Cheng became a great teacher because he was a superior student. He made the most of Yang's square while cultivating his own level and plumb. A dancer must not look like a puppet of the choreographer, but the inventor of the dance, and not only the inventor, but the inventor at the moment of performance. Cheng used the traditional metaphor, "fuel and fire," to describe the process of transmission from teacher to student. We might extend this by saying that a pure flame is capable of igniting both crude and refined fuel and likewise an impure flame. A pure flame can burn off impurities in crude fuel to produce another pure flame, and even an impure flame touching very refined fuel can produce a pure flame. Yang Ch'eng-fu was perhaps the purest and most powerful fuel of his day, and surely Cheng Man-ch'ing was the most refined fuel. His flame in turn has brought the art one step closer to the *tao* and given us a glimpse of what Chuang Tzu called, "riding on the laws of the universe."

Prof. Douglas Wile
Brooklyn College
Winter, 1985

BIOGRAPHY OF MAN-JAN
[CHENG MAN-CH'ING]

In my youth I went to school near Mt. K'uang-lu[1] and during my free time visited all the old Buddhist temples there. At the Hai-hui Temple I met an old monk from Hopei who was about eighty years old. He never ate after twelve o'clock noon and his complexion was like a child's. He was also a master of the martial arts. The back of the temple faced the Five Old Peaks, and a kind of edible fungus grew on the sheer cliffs. No one else was able to reach them, but the old monk went gathering often. Pulling himself up with the aid of pine trees and vines, he displayed the ease of an agile monkey or a bird in flight. Such was the lightness of his body.

Later I visited Mt. Ch'ing-ch'eng[2] and met Taoist Master Hung at the Ch'ang-tao Monastery. He was close to seventy years old. I noticed that at night he repaired to a wooden bed, and without quilt or pillow, sat regulating his breath. He said that this had been his practice for forty years. His hair and beard were black as lacquer and his voice was resonant.

If I were to count the number of extraordinary men I have met in my life, Man-jan would be the third. As a child he was high-spirited and playful. He followed his inclinations wherever they led him. He was intelligent and sensitive, reacting immediately to events. One day while playing near a dangerous wall, it collapsed injuring his head. When he regained consciousness, his mental faculties were somewhat diminished. Later, too, he contracted tuberculosis. However, after studying T'ai-chi ch'üan, his mind returned to normal and his physical condition daily improved. After a number of years, even those of imposing physique seemed weak

when compared to Man-jan. He showed an equal ap-
titude for classical studies, medicine, painting and calligraphy. He was also fond of travel, and no scenic
landscape or secluded valley was too inaccessible.
Once he encountered a tiger, but was undaunted, for
he had great inner strength and never showed fear. He
was an excellent physician and explained that drugs
could only control disease, but T'ai-chi ch'üan could
eliminate it. How can a nation of sick people avoid
humiliation? Although we possess the weapons of war,
without strong soldiers to wield them, we might as
well be totally unarmed. Confucius' teaching was based
on the Six Arts, but without training in archery and
charioteering, there would be no opportunity to pursue
rites, music, calligraphy or mathematics.

Our habits and customs are different from those
of Westerners. Therefore, there must be a form of exercise for achieving health which is appropriate to our
people. The choice is T'ai-chi ch'üan. This was Man-jan's
conviction and he communicated it untiringly to
everyone he met. His students numbered nearly ten
thousand. With this kind of interest, he was concerned
that the benefits reach the great masses of people. It
was for this reason that he wrote *Master Cheng's Thirteen Chapters on T'ai-chi Ch'üan*. He has carefully sur-
veyed his subject and clearly set forth its principles.
Withholding nothing, he has revealed the secrets of
the past and the essence of his own experience.

Sun Tzu's Art of War[3] has come down to us in
thirteen chapters. Although its authenticity has not been
established, it is indispensable for students of military
strategy. In titling his work on T'ai-chi ch'üan the *"Thirteen Chapters"* was it not his intention that it serve as
a foundation for military strategists and a guide for
statesmen? The world is in great travail and our nation
is still without peace. Thus Man-jan's purpose becomes

apparent. He regarded mountain top monastics and pious self-cultivators as withdrawing from the life and death struggle of the nation and as careless of the course of world events.

Man-jan was a native of Yung-chia County, Chekiang. His family name was Cheng, his given name Yüe, and his style, Man-ch'ing. Long ago, Chu-ko Liang[4] praised Kuan Chuang-mou's[5] sideburns [*jan*] as setting him apart from the common. Following this example, he took "jan" as his name.

Min Hsia-chi of Chiuchiang, Kiangsi Province.

AUTHOR'S PREFACE

In my youth I suffered from incurable beriberi and rheumatism. After practicing the exercises in the *Sinew Changing Classic,*[1] I improved. As a young man I also contracted tuberculosis, spitting up blood and coughing uncontrollably. After practicing T'ai-chi ch'üan, again I improved. In my younger days I was foolish, and as soon as my illness improved, I abandoned the exercises. After contracting tuberculosis, I realized that my constitution was weak. Of what use was wearying myself with practice? Looking at my past and at my future, I was overcome with grief. However, to my surprise, after practicing for only a few months, my illness completely disappeared. I therefore concluded that nothing was more efficacious for me than this martial art. How could I abandon it? I came to see it as more important than even food or sleep.

To this very day I have practiced without fail for seven minutes every morning after rising and in the evening before retiring. I am full of energy and daily advance towards perfect health. As precious as this is, I dare not keep it secret, but desire to present the fruits of my many years of experience to the martial artists and athletes of the world today. Both the principles and practice of T'ai-chi ch'üan have unique features which cannot be matched by any other martial art or exercise. Those who studied this art in the past either boasted of extraordinary powers or cultivated only themselves. As a result, the path became narrower and narrower. Thus it is that the superior man is never too self-satisfied. Today I understand Vimalakirti's compassion for the sick[2] and vow to live up to Confucius' capacity for empathy. In the spirit of "sharing the good with others"[3] so that it reaches the whole world, I desire to help the weak become strong and the sickly well and active. This being my purpose, how could I be dilatory in the writing of this book?

My teacher, Yang Ch'eng-fu, suspended the family transmission. He did not lightly share his knowledge, fearing that it would fall into the wrong hands. Therefore only the outline of his principles and applications has been transmitted to the world. At the request of myself and fellow student, K'uang K'o-ming, Yang's book was published in May of 1934.[4] At the time my own understanding was very superficial and I did not appreciate how great were its benefits to mankind. Now Master Yang has already passed away, and though we desire to receive more of what he had to offer, it is impossible to obtain. For this reason I have taken all of these secrets and presented them in this book. My hope is to promote the principles of the great physicians of old who treated the people before they became ill, and sharing this with the world's true seekers, demonstrate that *ch'i* cultivation is the basis of self-strengthening and hence of national salvation. May my people rise again!

Preface written by Cheng Man-ch'ing of Yung-chia during the Double Nine Festival[5] in Nanking, 1946.

CHAPTER

1

THE MEANING OF "T'AI-CHI"

Martial arts are a form of exercise which combine principle and practice and increase both wisdom and courage. T'ai-chi is the mother of *yin* and *yang* and all-embracing in its scope. To thus name a martial art is of profound significance. The *I ching* states that T'ai-chi gives birth to the two aspects: *yin* and *yang*.[1] When *yin* reaches its peak, it produces *yang*; when *yang* reaches its peak, it produces *yin*. The dynamic processes of hard and soft, movement and stasis, are all based on these peaks.

The strong are fond of using the martial arts for combat. Victory or defeat in combat is their standard for judging one's level of skill in martial arts. Those who love combat never fail to use stiff and brutish force to strike their opponents, or fast techniques to grapple with them. This is the peak of *yang*, the extreme of hardness. If one's defense against this is hard, the result will be defeat and injury for both parties. This is not mastery. If my opponent uses hardness, I neutralize it with softness. If my opponent attacks with movement, I meet him with stillness. The height of softness and stillness is the peak of *yin*. When the peak of *yang* encounters the peak of *yin*, the *yang* is invariably defeated. This is what Lao Tzu referred to as softness and weakness overcoming hardness and strength.[2] Therefore, let me say that to study T'ai-chi ch'üan, one must begin by "investing in loss." At its highest level, learning to invest in loss produces precisely its opposite. This is the ultimate in gaining the position of advantage. We may compare this to the teeth, which are firm and hard, and the tongue, which is soft. Occasionally the teeth and tongue have disagreements, and the tongue must temporarily invest in loss, but in the end the teeth will crumble from hardness, while the tongue will survive through softness. This illustrates my meaning.

Those who pursue the martial arts always seek to overcome others and gain the advantage. Today, who is willing to learn investment in loss? It must be understood that investment in loss means allowing others to attack us with force, while we do not use the slightest strength to resist. Rather, we attract this force and deflect it, allowing it to dissipate into nothingness so that its effect is completely lost. Thus, with the slightest release of our hands, the opponent is invariably thrown for a great distance. This is what the T'ai-chi classics call "interpreting energy." They state, "After learning to interpret energy, it can be perfected to the point that one can straightaway accomplish whatever the mind desires."[3] This is the height of gaining the advantage. Moreover, the subtlety and marvelous applications of this art correspond at every point with the principle of the Great Ultimate (T'ai-chi). Beginning with Chang San-feng, it has been transmitted without interruption "as fire springs from fuel"[4] with "each generation preserving the best."[5] Only after receiving the spiritual transmission of T'ai-chi ch'üan from Yang Ch'eng-fu, did I begin to appreciate that its application was entirely based on the Great Ultimate. The truth of the mutual production of *yin* and *yang* and the mutual destruction of hard and soft can all be demonstrated in practice. Thus there is good reason for calling this art the "Great Ultimate." Not only are its practitioners able to neutralize hardness and speed and enjoy first place among the martial arts, but it strengthens the weak, raises the sick, invigorates the debilitated, and encourages the timid. Truly it is the way of strengthening the individual, the race, and the nation. Can our leaders who seek to alleviate the suffering of the people afford to overlook this?

CHAPTER

2

UNDERSTANDING THE MYSTERIOUS AND THE SUBSTANTIAL

The term "T'ai-chi" appears in the *Book of Changes (I ching)*[1] and is also found in the Chinese medical classics[2] and the *Taoist Canon (Tao tsang)*.[3] Its theory is broad and its applications unlimited, or what Confucious called, "embracing all of the transformations in Heaven and earth without error."[4] Its principles are all contained within *yin* and *yang*; the transformations of its *ch'i* are all explained by the Five Phases.[5] This is the embryo of our nation's culture and philosophy. To abandon *yin* and *yang* and the Five Phases in discussing T'ai-chi is to engage in baseless nonsense, unworthy of serious consideration. If one insists on disregarding *yin* and *yang* and the Five Phases in discussing Chinese philosophy, medicine, or Taoism, one might as well ignore addition, subtraction, multiplication, division, and algebra in discussing mathematics. Is this possible?

Today, scientific progress is such that we have now advanced from the electrical to the atomic age. However, allow me to ask if it is possible to depart from the function of *yin* and *yang*? T'ai-chi ch'üan is in accord with philosophy and science, for its theory is purely philosophical and its attitude completely scientific. This can be demonstrated through its actual principles and practice and does not require skillful rhetoric. However, the original writings on T'ai-chi ch'üan are exceedingly subtle and their practice truly extraordinary. For the moment, let us confine ourselves to general concepts and analyze just a few examples. In terms of movement, when they speak of "using the mind to direct the *ch'i,* and the *ch'i* to mobilize the body,"[6] it is always the case that movement follows mobilization. This is like an electric train or steamship which borrows the power of *ch'i* and mobilizes it to produce motion. How completely unlike merely moving the limbs or isolated parts of the body, and calling this movement.[7] Also, what we call "relaxation of the abdomen," "light-ness and sensitivity of the whole body," and "using four ounces to repel a thousand pounds" are all said to require no strength.[8] Those who do not use strength cannot be the object of the strength of an opponent's attack, and thus they maintain the controlling position. This is the essential principle and is relatively simple. To repel a thousand pounds with four ounces is the application. How can a thousand pounds be repelled with four ounces? By determining our opponent's center of gravity and causing him to lean to one side, without even applying four ounces to repel him, he will topple by himself. In presenting these kinds of principles to the athletes of the world, we should prefer to emphasize its correspondence with philosophy or science. Beyond this, there is what we call the concen-tration of *ch'i* in the bones.[9] When this reaches the point where the bones achieve "essential hardness,"[10] "there is nothing that can stand up to them."[11] To explain this any further is simply a waste of words.

In the spring of 1929, Mr. Ts'ao Chung, a student of electrical engineering, was interested in learning something of the art of T'ai-chi ch'üan from me. I spoke to him about sinking the *ch'i* to the *tan-t'ien,* and he asked of what advantage this was. I replied that sinking the *ch'i* to the *tan-t'ien* was surely beneficial, but not nearly so much as maintaining both the mind and the *ch'i* in the *tan-t'ien.* There was absolutely nothing more beneficial to the body than this. He desired a more detailed explanation, and I continued by saying that the abdomen contains the largest concentration of water in the body. In the external environment the harmful effects of water result on a large scale in major floods or on a small scale in breaching dikes and levees, as well as high water and excessive rain. In the human body, a great excess produces abdominal distension, jaundice, or "damp-blockage;"[12] a lesser excess results in phlegm and excessive fluid, ulcerated sores, or scabies together with damp-heat and sultry summer-heat conditions afflicting the lungs, spleen, stomach and intestines. There are too many examples to enumerate. To dispel these water related illnesses, nothing is as effective as exercise. The Emperor Yü[13] succeeded in controlling the floods by dredging the waterways and channeling the water. It is also very much like the process in nature of sunlight evaporating water, dispelling the darkness, and reducing clouds and rain. If this can be duplicated in the human body, then it can be said that we have stolen the secret power of Heaven.

How is it that simply concentrating the mind and *ch'i* in the *tan-t'ien* can produce such a definite effect? Sinking the *ch'i* is like introducing hot air into a wine jar with the effect of dispelling dampness and cold. When *ch'i* and the mind are maintained together in the *tan-t'ien,* it is like placing fire beneath a pot which causes the water inside to boil and gradually turn to steam. This is not only perfectly safe, but very beneficial to the blood circulation. Its effectiveness is truly remarkable! Mr. Ts'ao responded by exclaiming, "How wonderful! I have always considered philosophy to be simply philosophy, but now I realize that philosophy is the science of the future." I added that there was an even more advanced level. When *ch'i* "collects in the bones,"[14] they acquire "essential hardness,"[15] that is to say, *ch'i* passes from the *tan-t'ien* through the *wei-lü* point and ascends the spinal column. When Mr. Ts'ao heard this, he was very amazed and repeated it to a Western doctor who replied that he was familiar with a phenomenon closely related to the idea of sinking *ch'i* to the *tan-t'ien*. He said that recently a French doctor, while dissecting a cadaver, had discovered a sort of pocket amidst the membranes connecting the intestines in the abdomen. Only in athletes was this pocket well developed. If one used a fist or rod to strike them, this pocket could be raised or lowered to withstand the blow. Perhaps what the Chinese call the *tan-t'ien* is the same as this pocket.

Mr. Ts'ao responded by saying that there was no path from the *wei-lü* point up the spine, and hence nothing could pass through. I answered that his knowledge was limited by his own experience and that he was not willing to seek further. What has been described as a specially developed pocket in athletes, and their ability to manipulate it to withstand blows, is indeed true. What this pocket contains is none other than *ch'i*. When one has accumulated a great deal of *ch'i*, it passes through the membranes. These membranes must naturally be more developed than most people's, and not only can they be raised or lowered to withstand blows, but forwards and backwards, to the left and right, as well. It is *ch'i* which has permeated the membranes and not the pocket itself which moves up and down in self-defense. If there was a direct path, then all would be aware of it, and this knowledge would not be so rare.

When the mind and *ch'i* are both concentrated in the *tan-t'ien*, not only can water be transmuted into *ch'i*, but *ching*[15] can also be transmuted into *ch'i*. In transmuting *ching* into *ch'i*, the heat of the *ch'i* can be compared to electricity, which is able to pass through water, earth, and metals without difficulty. How much more easily from the *wei-lü* up the spine! The *wei-lü* and spine have many joints, and although there is no direct path, they are not without their vital points. Having these vital points, there must be a passageway which is simply a connection formed of sinews and cartilage. First we isolate these vital points and heat them with the *ching-ch'i*[17] and the heart's fire, augmenting this with the *ch'i* of the *tan-t'ien*. Then we stir it up and set it in motion, causing the *ching-ch'i* to be converted into heat which passes through the *wei-lü* up the spine, reaching the crown of the head and spreading out to the four limbs. This further causes the warm *ch'i* to condense in the bones, where it is sealed in and cannot issue forth. In a short time the *ch'i* transmuted from *ching* once again reverts to water, and then gradually to fatty fluid. The fatty fluid then becomes solid matter in the form of bone marrow which sticks to the inside of the bones. This is very much like the process of nickel or gold plating, or what the ancients called, "daily progress by the thickness of one sheet of paper." This is precisely what they were referring to. After a long time, the marrow becomes very full, and the bones firm and strong. This is why we refer to them as "essentially hard." Their ability to "smash even the hardest object"[18] is a result of the process just described.

All of this may be attained without departing from the principles of *yin* and *yang* and the Five Phases. But there is an even further proof. My teacher, Yang Ch'eng-fu's arms were at least ten times heavier than an ordinary person's. When he used them to attack, none could resist. Though I myself have not reached the level of my teacher, my arms are several times heavier than most peoples'. This may be verified. Now a tiger's bones are different from those of other animals. This is because they are filled with rock-like marrow which is without the slightest gap. Therefore, they are exceptionally strong. This may also be verified. However, it is but one example of T'ai-chi ch'üan's correspondence with philosophy and science. Mr. Ts'ao responded, "Oh, how wonderful! T'ai-chi ch'üan has its origins in philosophy and is verified by science. Your words are very true." I answered that what I had described was simply the alchemical transmutation of *ching* into *ch'i* and the transformation of *ch'i* to "fortify the brain."[19] But there is a still more advanced level. When the *ching* has been transmuted into *ch'i,* the *ch'i* is then transmuted into spirit, which reverts to emptiness and reaches a state of supremely subtle sensitivity. This is beyond my own attainment. Mr. Ts'ao replied, "Say no more! I understand your meaning. If the principle exists, then the reality must necessarily follow. But let us leave the proof for another day."

3

CONCENTRATING THE *CH'I* AND DEVELOPING SOFTNESS

T'ai-chi ch'üan's special advantage lies in sinking the *ch'i* to the *tan-t'ien*. Sinking the *ch'i* is the first phase of training in what Lao Tzu called, "Concentrating the *ch'i* and developing softness."[1] From Lao Tzu's phrase, "The soft and weak are the followers of life; the hard and strong are the followers of death,"[2] we can see that the way of cultivating life lies in becoming soft. If we desire to develop softness, we must first pay attention to concentrating the *ch'i*. Concentrating the *ch'i* can be said to have "arrived at its highest good"[3] in the *tan-t'ien*. The sinking of the *ch'i* to the *tan-tien* is expressed in the *I ching* when it says, "Water over fire represents completion." In hexagram 63, "After Completion" ䷾ the trigrams representing fire and water mutually interact. This hexagram consists of the trigrams *K'an* ☵ and *Li* ☲   *Li* is the fire of the heart (mind)[4] which rises like flames; *K'an* is the water of the kidneys[5] which flows downward. If allowed to turn their backs on each other and gallop off in the spirit of hardness and strength, then this is precisely the opposite of becoming soft.

In human beings the abdomen contains the largest amount of water, about 70 per cent. There are two fires:[6] that of the ruler and that of the prime minister.[7] In the *I ching's* "Sequence of Later Heaven" *Li* is the fire of the ruler,[8] that is, the heart's (mind's) fire which is substantial fire. [9] The fire in what the *Classic of Inter-*

nal Medicine calls the *ming-men*[10] is the fire of the prime minister, or empty fire.[11] The Five Viscera and Six Bowels,[12] as well as the whole body, rely on the fanning of the two fires, ruler and minister. There is no place that the fire cannot reach. An excess of fire results in illness. This is what Chinese medicine means when it says that such and such a place "has fire," or what Western medicine calls "inflammation." Thus it is apparent that, although fire is diffused throughout the body, it does not diminish the accumulation of the power of water. If the human body lacks water, then it quickly becomes dehydrated. If it lacks fire, then the power of digestion will be affected. Not only are deficiencies of water and fire undesirable, but excesses as well. If given free rein, then one rises and the other sinks, which the *I ching* calls "Before Completion."[13] Can this be sustained for very long?

Lao Tzu read the *I ching* and apprehended its true meaning. Following its principles he said, "Concentrate your *ch'i* and develop softness," which is the method of sinking the *ch'i* to the *tan-t'ien* and maintaining it there together with the mind. The *tan-t'ien* is the stove of the *tan* elixir.[14] When the mind is within the stove and the water is on top, the fire heats the water, and rather than suffering the ill effects of water sinking, we benefit from the marvel of its transmutation into *ch'i* (steam). When water is above and water below, water completes fire. In this way, not only are we spared the danger of fire's rising, but enjoy the natural process of warming and sustaining. This is called "After Completion,"[15] with the trigrams *K'an* above and *Li* below. It indicates the fulfillment of concentrating the *ch'i* and developing softness, or not allowing water and fire to violate the *tao*.

Some say they understand the idea that water above and fire below represents "After Completion," but ask why it is necessary to first concentrate the *ch'i* in order to become soft. I say that nothing is more beneficial than concentrating the *ch'i*. Let me discuss for a moment some of the most important aspects of this. First, the *tan-t'ien* is simply like a pocket of *ch'i*. If we do not sink our *ch'i* to the *tan-t'ien*, then the pocket will collapse and close up. In this condition, although the *tan-t'ien* is present, it is useless. Even if we desire to mobilize the heart's fire and direct it to the *tan-t'ien*, it will be impossible. Secondly, if the mind and *ch'i* are not connected, then everything will be unfocused and there will be nowhere to direct the mind-force. How will we know if it has reached the *tan-t'ien* or not? Therefore, in sinking the concentrated *ch'i* to the *tan-t'ien*, it is especially important that the mind be maintained there as well. Only then can we achieve softness. This is what the "Treatise on T'ai-chi ch'üan" calls, "moving the *ch'i* with the mind," "moving the body with the *ch'i*," and "*ch'i* filling the whole body." Without exception, the *ch'i* must first sink to the *tan-t'ien*, and only then can we speak of the ability to mobilize or move the *ch'i*. This is only one aspect of the function of concentrating the *ch'i*.

Some may ask, now that we understand what is meant by concentrating the *ch'i*, what are the full benefits to the human body? Our answer is that this has already been explained by Lao Tzu when he says, "In concentrating your *ch'i* and becoming soft, can you be like an infant?"[16] An infant is like the sprouting seed of a human being. Because the expression of the life-force has not yet been suspended, it is soft and weak like the sprouts of grass and trees. When it is mature and approaching old age, it no longer expresses the life-force and becomes hard and strong. This is like the strong tree which easily breaks. It is not far from death. Can those people who are not far from death return to the state of infancy? The infant's body is pure *yang*. Pure *yang* means that the *ch'i* is abundant. When the *ch'i* is abundant, the blood is sufficient and the sinews are soft. Soft sinews are a special characteristic of the infant. If people who are not far from death are to have any hope of returning to youthfulness, it is only through concentrating the *ch'i* and becoming soft. If we are to be saved from the mad waves after capsizing or preserve our mental faculties which are about to be annihilated, then it can only be through the power of fire under water, as in the hexagram "After Completion."

Let me now speak of the final stage. The T'ai chi ch'üan classics begin by saying, "The *ch'i* should be roused and the spirit gathered within," and end with, "Our consciousness should be on the spirit and not on the *ch'i*. If our consciousness is on the *ch'i*, then it is blocked. If there is *ch'i* then there is no strength; without *ch'i* essential hardness is achieved."[17] From this it becomes comprehensible. "Rousing" means that one's own *ch'i* and the atmosphere interact. This is a step beyond "mobilizing the *ch'i*, moving the *ch'i*, and *ch'i* filling the whole body." "Gathering the spirit" is an even more advanced level of the power of concentrating the *ch'i*. The height of concentrating the *ch'i* is the ability to transmute *ching* into *ch'i*. However, even transmuting *ching* into *ch'i* is not yet at the stage of pure undifferentiated *yang*. As for "keeping one's consciousness on the spirit and not on the *ch'i*," and "without *ch'i* then essential hardness is achieved," this is the ultimate, the culmination. T'ai-chi ch'üan can reach the stage of pure undifferentiated *yang*,[18] which corresponds from beginning to end with Lao Tzu's theory of concentrating the *ch'i* and developing softness. If we are able to achieve this, then the theory of eliminating illness and prolonging life is simply a logical extension.

CHAPTER

4

TRANSFORMING ONE'S DISPOSITION

To read the works of the Sages and great men, to diligently practice, to examine, to carefully ponder and clearly discriminate, this at its highest level is what is called, "making the Six Classics[1] a footnote to oneself." I have no doubt that this can lead to the transformation of one's disposition. As for the study of T'ai-chi ch'üan also having the ability to transform the disposition, this I have never heard of. I have practiced T'ai-chi ch'üan for thirty years, and continuously without interruption for twenty-one, but I myself do not know if my disposition has been transformed. I respectfully relate my own experience for those of greater wisdom to judge.

In my youth, although possessed of the potential for righteousness and courage, I was reckless and belligerent. I took risks with my life without the slightest care. I loved study and strove for perfection, but my physical strength and spirit were not equal to it. As a result, I often stopped in mid-course and changed direction, without ever accomplishing anything. Now I am already approaching old age; what more is there to say. Nevertheless, I have never cared for comforts, wealth, or honor, but only to know the way (*tao*) "which when heard in the morning one can die peacefully at night."[2] Perhaps this is worthy of admiration, so I did not give in to "self-destructiveness or despair."[3]

Having studied T'ai-chi ch'üan for the past twenty odd years, what I have personally witnessed is its ability

to rouse the infirm, raise the weak, and eliminate illness. This much I have already achieved and can maintain it for a long time without flagging. As for stopping
in mid-course and changing direction, perhaps there
has been some reform. When it comes to the attainment
of inner peace and serenity, however, I dare not make
such claims. Nevertheless, my former recklessness and
belligerence have perhaps been somewhat eliminated.
To speak though of transforming my disposition would
be like attempting to transform brambles into orchids
or owls into phoenixes. I dare not aspire to this.

I believe that those whose spirit and physical
strength are deficient, even if they are young and strong
will become weak and sick. When weakness and disease
assail us, no matter how we strive to improve ourselves,
we cannot succeed, much less transform our disposi-
tions. Not being able to improve themselves, people
engage in efforts to cling to youth or tranquility, acting
like pampered wives, beautiful concubines, or effemi-
nate boys. So we can understand why traitors or corrupt
officials who know they cannot succeed in their crimes,
commit them anyway. For this reason, I know that most
people would rather be whole tiles than fragments of
jade.[4] I am afraid that half the people have not sufficient
strength or spirit to sustain themselves. This discussion
of transforming one's disposition applies only to per-
sons of normal endowment. To approach it is to gradually become a superior man; to fall away from it is to
gradually become an inferior man. Therefore I say
when asked if T'ai-chi ch'üan is able to transform the
disposition, that this must await demonstration by one
wiser than myself.

5

SWIMMING
ON DRY LAND

The softest of all exercises is swimming. This is recognized today by scholars of all nations. Thus it can be seen that softness is the most marvelous method of exercise. However, the disadvantages of swimming are many. For example, one may contract such contagious diseases as trachoma and gonorrhea or infections from water entering the throat, ears, and nose. In the case of those with weak hearts, drowning may even occur. I need not go on, but these are the shortcomings of swimming. Nevertheless, swimming has two unique advantages: one in principle and one in practice. In principle it allows us to become strong swimmers; in practice it promotes stamina. Those who are good swimmers and have great stamina show the results of the function of *ch'i*.

Strong swimmers must have the ability to hold the breath. The longer we are able to hold the breath the more we improve as swimmers. Stamina is also a function of the ability to hold the breath. The longer one can hold the breath, the greater the volume of breath. Increasing the volume of breath represents an advance in the power of *ch'i*. What we refer to as stamina is simply the development of *ch'i*. Therefore, those who are strong swimmers and have also developed their *ch'i* invariably excel at floating. Thus if we combine the special advantages of both principle and practice, would this not be called softness? This is what Lao Tzu referred to as the method of concentrating the *ch'i* and developing softness. That which distinguishes T'ai-chi ch'üan from other exercises is simply that its special advantage lies in concentrating the *ch'i* and developing softness. From this point of view, swimming cannot compare to T'ai-chi ch'üan. From the point of view of increasing stamina without attendant dangers, T'ai-chi ch'üan is also far superior to swimming.

T'ai-chi ch'üan is also called "Long Boxing," or as it is said, "slow and continuous like great rivers and seas."[1] This perfectly describes the idea of unbroken motion. Unbroken motion is nothing other than concentrating the *ch'i* and developing softness. This is precisely the same as the way one functions in swimming. The reason why fish excel at swimming is that they are born and raised in water. Does this mean that they understand the function of water? The reason why human beings excel at walking is that they were born and raised in air. But they do not understand the function of air. Nevertheless, if fish are removed from water they die, and if human beings are removed from air, their life ceases. In this respect they are the same. Thus, while water and air are not the same, the need for them is one. Although human beings and fish are not the same, their response to removal from their element is identical. From this we may conclude that what air is to human beings, water is to fish. My swimming on dry land, or imagining that I am swimming, then becomes perfectly possible. For this reason I have created the concept of swimming on dry land.

Human beings live on dry land and while they are actually swimming in air, they have been unaware of it for a long time. How much more so the function of this air? Oh, how great indeed is air! There is nothing it does not contain, nothing it does not envelop. This is truly supreme! In its functioning, there is nothing it does not support, nothing it does not nourish. We know it is thus, but we do not know the reason. The teachings of the Yellow Emperor,[2] Ch'i Po, [3] and Lao Tzu are revelations so subtle and detailed that we can never exhaust them. Some people do not have the strength to tie up a chicken, and some can carry a great caldron. They are both human beings, but how can they be so far apart in their strength?

The source of strength is connected with *ch'i*. Those whose strength is great have strong *ch'i*. Strong *ch'i* is the result of storing *ch'i*. Storing *ch'i* is like storing water. If the store of water is shallow, there will be little buoyancy and even a cup or a plate will not easily float. When the store of water is deeper, then a ten ton ship will seem to float weightlessly. Those who are able to carry great caldrons simply possess a somewhat deeper store of *ch'i*. If we could only realize that the secret of storing *ch'i* is like storing water, then our strength would be infinite and lifting a great caldron would seem a trifling feat.

Storing *ch'i* means storing it in the *tan-t'ien*. The *tan-t'ien* is the "Sea of Ch'i" (*ch'i-hai*), and is located 1.3 inches below the navel. Comparing it to the sea allows us to understand its capacity, sustaining power, immensity and depth. There is nothing else to it. If *ch'i* reverts to the "sea" and accumulates for days and months without interruption, after three years one will be able to see significant progress. Now this is nothing more than stealing the *ch'i* of Heaven and earth for ourselves, like one hair from a herd of ten thousand cattle. How does one begin the work of storing *ch'i* to achieve this result? Our answer is that T'ai-chi ch'üan is the method for storing *ch'i* and the technique for circulating it. With this it overflows into the sinews, reaches the bone marrow, fills the membranes and diaphragm, and manifests in the hair and skin. This is truly concentrating the *ch'i* and developing softness.

The exercise for concentrating the *ch'i* and developing softness which most closely corresponds to the principles of T'ai-chi ch'üan is swimming. If we expend one minute's worth of strength, then we see the results of one minute's worth of strength; if we expend a quarter of an hour's worth of effort then we see the results of a quarter of an hour's worth of effort. Our progress will be steady over the days and months. But precisely because it cannot be measured, therefore I use it as a comparison for T'ai-chi ch'üan. Students can use objective phenomena as models to facilitate understanding. Air is not empty; it is just like water. With every movement we feel the turbulence of the air, just as if we were swimming. Inhaling, exhaling, floating and sinking, as well as moving forwards and backwards, are all like swimming. If we can attain this level, we have already gone beyond the ordinary person. Beginners can start by simply moving their hands or stretching out their limbs in the wind in order to realize that wind and air are similar to water. At the highest level, we become aware that air is not only heavier than water, but even iron.

That air is heavier than iron is a new scientific discovery related to me a long time ago by my friend, Mr. Ts'ao Chung. He said that in experiments where air was introduced under intense pressure into an iron container, and used as an explosive device, its power exceeded that of conventional bombs. I was skeptical, and to this day cannot explain it. However, since the invention of the atomic bomb, the idea that air is heavier than iron is not so strange after all. The movements of T'ai-chi ch'üan flow from the storing of *ch'i*. Its power to support weight is even greater than that of water. This, then, is the truth of the ability of concentrating *ch'i* and developing softness to overcome great hardness. If we work with the concept of swimming in air, we will "surely receive great benefit."[4]

6

THE EQUAL IMPORTANCE
OF HEART AND SPINE

The *Classic of Internal Medicine* speaks of the *Jen* and *Tu* meridians together. Other ancient works also refer to the heart (mind) and spine together, and the Taoists are most explicit about the relationship between the heart and spine and self-cultivation. T'ai-chi ch'üan is an internal system. The Immortal Chang San-feng,[1] who lived at the end of the Sung dynasty [960-1126], followed the Yellow Emperor and Lao Tzu's theory of action arising from non-action, combined with the *I ching's* concepts of principle (*li*), *ch'i,* and image (*hsiang*)[2] as the basis for his development. Fundamentally, this is none other than the *Jen* and *Tu* meridians. The *Jen* and *Tu* are the most important of the Eight Extra Channels (*ch'i-ching pa-mai*).[3] The *Jen* is ruled by the heart, the *Tu* by the spine. The spine is associated with the kidneys. In terms of distinguishing them according to essence and function, the spine is essence and the heart is function. In terms of their unity, when heart and kidneys interact properly, then essence and function are complete. The reason why T'ai-chi ch'üan surpasses all other martial arts or exercises is because of its attention to this.

The heart is the ruler of the whole body. The core of the learning of the Sages and wise men may be summarized in the words, "Reclaim our true hearts."[4] Ch'an Buddhists say, "Is the master at home?" The master is the heart. This is virtually identical with the Taoist emphasis on the proper interaction between heart and kidneys. These are simply different approaches to the same end, and each arrives at its proper place. Only T'ai-chi ch'üan takes a step beyond this. This is precisely what is meant by nothing being more profound or clear than when it is actually demonstrated in practice. For this reason I have advanced the theory of the equal importance of heart and spine with the hope of revealing the truth that where there is principle there must also be application.

The heart is not the lump of flesh known as the heart, but the spiritual heart. The spiritual heart and the heart of flesh were not originally two, but also not one. That is to say, the reason why the heart which is flesh is able to function, and more subtly than anything else, is because of the spiritual heart. The "spine" refers to the backbone. The spine has twenty-four joints. It is the most important bone in the human body and has the greatest number of joints. The internal organs are all attached to it; the Five Appendages[5] and trunk depend upon it for support. However, this is of secondary importance, for in speaking of self-cultivation or health to ignore the spine is to be completely superficial. Herein lies T'ai-chi ch'üan's devotion to the root.

Beginners must maintain both mind and *ch'i* in the *tan-t'ien*. They must neither "forget this nor force it."[6] This is what is known as "reclaiming our true minds,"[7] or the master being at home. After a long time, the *ch'i* naturally travels to the *wei-lü*, rushes through the *chia-chi*, traverses the *yü-chen*, and finally reaches the crown of the head from which it descends again to the *tan-t'ien*.[8] This, then, is the connection of the *Jen* and *Tu* meridians, and the interaction of the heart and kidneys. However this is not the work of one day; it cannot be forced and must be completely natural. If one can achieve it, then not only is there hope of

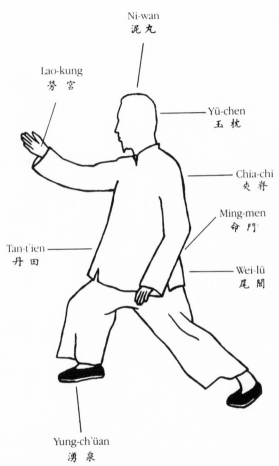

Ni-wan
泥 丸

Lao-kung
勞 宮

Yü-chen
玉 枕

Chia-chi
夾 脊

Ming-men
命 門

Tan-t'ien
丹 田

Wei-lü
尾 閭

Yung-ch'üan
湧 泉

reaching the pinnacle of perfection in T'ai-chi ch'üan, but immortality of the spirit, long life and health as well.

The mind is a difficult thing to discuss, though there has been no shortage of scholars and spiritual seekers who have tried. For example, we have the ancient philosophical theories of "the mental transmission of teachings," "rectification of the mind," and "the imperturbability of the mind."[9] Truly these principles, as eternal as "the passage of the sun and the moon in the heavens" may serve as our model; what need for further explanations? However, the meaning of the one word, "spine," has not yet been fully elucidated. In general, what the ancients called, "straightening the lapels and sitting precariously,"[10] refers to the process of self-cultivation. Explanations of the word "precarious" are many, but none have dared to relate it directly to the idea of danger. I believe that "sitting precariously" contains within it the actual element of danger. The spine has many joints, just like a string of pearls, rising one on top of the other. If we are heedless for an instant and lean to one side or bend over, then we no longer have the strength to support the trunk. In terms of illness, this may result in bone ulcers, tubercles, or even damage to the cervical vertebrae. Is this not dangerous? Those who excel at self-cultivation, understanding this, do not allow themselves to gradually become lethargic and fall into illness. Therefore, as a warning to those treading on loose footing near a great precipice, it is said, "straighten the lapels and sit precariously." If one is straight, there will be no illness; if precarious, then one will be cautious of deviating from the straight with the result of illness. Therefore, I advise practitioners of T'ai-chi ch'üan to straighten their spines. Holding the spine erect is like stringing pearls one on top of the other, without letting them lean or incline. However, if one is tense and stiff, or unnaturally affected, then this too is an error. All we need do is be aware of the danger and that should be sufficient.

CHAPTER

7

ENERGY AND PHYSICS

The application of *ch'i* and energy (*chin*) in T'ai-chi ch'üan is slow and continuous, cyclical and repetitious, circular and inter-connected. It is inexhaustible. Within the universe, it is as great as the revolution of the planets and as fine as the droplets of rain or dew. Its forms are all round, a sign of its naturalness. To expand on this further, its essence, function, and subtle internal energy are all intimately related to the art of T'ai-chi ch'üan. Let us fully analyze this.

A planet is something so immense it seems that nothing could contain it. Because it is spherical, it can be supported by *ch'i* and is able to revolve. If its form were not spherical, then in spite of the power of *ch'i*, it could not be supported, nor could the countless stars be floated in space, all in revolution. Because it is round, its capacity is maximized and its surface area minimized. Even the finest drop of rain or dew contains infinite water molecules, each striving to expand outward. As a result, each remains in equilibrium because of their mutual attraction. While its surface is expansive, its center is cohesive, and therefore it does not lose its roundness. This then is the reason for roundness. T'ai-chi ch'üan's so called roundness comes from its imitating the Great Ultimate. The reason for this, as well as its essence and function, corresponds to the mystery of the natural world explained above. To illustrate this I have provided a diagram.

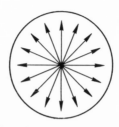

Looking at the above diagram, every point within the circumference of the circle is equidistant from the center. This is what Moh Tzu called "equal extension from a common center."[1] Furthermore, the resistance to stress on the circumference, whether the sphere is strong or weak, is equal at all points. Otherwise it could not maintain its spherical form. Thus a rubber ball and an iron ball are both spherical. Regardless of their weight, when force strikes their surface, we know that every point on the surface being equal, every point will move. Touch one point, and ten thousand points will respond. This is why in T'ai-chi ch'üan we do not allow an opponent to feel and touch us. Because our form is round, they cannot know where to apply their strength. When a sphere rotates, the mutual attraction of the molecules results in so called centripetal and centrifugal force.

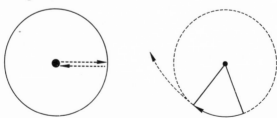

From the diagrams above, a force originating at the center and expanding outward is called centrifugal, and a force on the circumference drawn inward is called centripetal. If the two forces are not equal, the round form cannot be maintained. For example, let us attach a rock or a piece of iron to one end of a cord and hold the other end in our hand. If we twirl this around in a circle, then the hand is the center and the direction of force of the rock or piece of iron is outward. This is called centrifugal force. Because the pulling force of the cord is inward, it is called centripetal. At this point, even if the cord is not strong, we will be able to observe a vigorous force resulting from the tension. The strength of this force depends solely on the speed of the revolution. This, then, is the principle of T'ai-chi ch'üan Push-hands, or so called "sawing style" sparring. If the centripetal force received is very great, but is met with an equally great centrifugal force, then no matter how great the centripetal force, it can be neutralized. This is the result of practicing roundness. Moreover, because I meet him with centrifugal force, my opponent is unable to neutralize it and will be thrown for a great distance. However, this touches on only two points, centripetal and centrifugal force, which are but aspects of the function of roundness.

Beyond this, roundness also includes the function of squareness, for it contains an infinite number of equilateral triangles. The triangle is, in actuality, the basic form for the construction of the circle. (See figures below.)

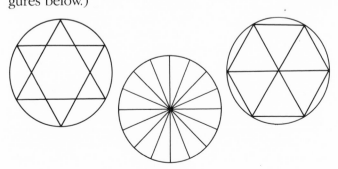

The function of the circle is intimately related to the triangles which it contains. In physics, applications of this can be seen in such inventions as the cone and the screw. From this we can see that the round form is not only strong and possessed of the negative defense function of resistance to external force, but because of the infinite triangles which it contains, can from any position apply positive attacking force. If we cause the sphere to rotate and press forward to attack, then there is not one square inch of surface that does not have the positive function of offense. This is similar to table tennis, where if one player attacks with a spinning ball, and the other player does not know the 'correct technique to respond, the attack cannot be withstood and defeat is inevitable. This is because of the short distance and speed of the attack which demonstrates the function of the circle containing infinite triangles. T'ai-chi ch'üan in relation to the circle described above maximizes the function of the infinite triangles, and its effectiveness is most dramatic. It takes roundness as a model, but is not really a sphere. Its defense is based on the principle of roundness; its offense is to be everywhere triangles. Moreover, there is not one inch which does not have the offensive potential of revolving triangles. This is why, when used to attack, the opponent will find it very difficult to escape. Beyond this, sometimes when on the offensive, one can transcend the function of the circle and suddenly transform it into an isosceles triangle, whose possibilities for application are even broader and whose attack is even fiercer. However, we have still not left the framework of the sphere.

From the following it can be seen that in T'ai-chi ch'üan every action is offensive and every point is defensive. This is what is meant by, "yielding is issuing and issuing is yielding." The positive is contained in the negative. This is also what is meant by, "My opponent

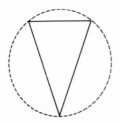 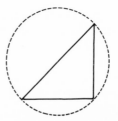

does not understand me, but I understand him. Wherever he goes the hero finds no equal."[2] What has been discussed above is the offensive function of circles containing infinite triangles. If, however, we should encounter a direct frontal attack which causes a concavity in the triangle, what then is the function? (See figure below.)

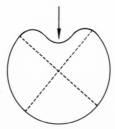

If we receive a direct attack without deviation to the left or right, up or down, then ignoring for the moment methods of escape to the left or right, up or down and simply addressing the attack itself, T'ai-chi ch'üan is able to actually exploit this fierce attack. This is why the *I ching* calls the trigram *K'an*, "entrapment,"[3] and why it is the most dangerous hexagram. It is also the first reason for naming this art, "T'ai-chi" (The Great Ultimate). The meaning is that it is able to cause outside aggression to land on nothing. When the opponent realizes that he has landed on nothing and is trapped, then he has no choice but to turn around and attempt to escape. Just as he seeks to extricate himself, then using the attractive force of my abdomen, I instantly apply repelling force. This is what writings on T'ai-chi ch'üan call "uprooting" (*t'i-fang*). "*Fang*" (release, put, shoot) means issuing energy and then once again returning to roundness. Thus the opponent has no time to act and is thrown for a great distance. This is T'ai-chi ch'üan's unique superiority: so called "issuing energy." The opposite is yielding, or also called transforming. Yielding is a rapid conversion; transforming is a slow conversion. Nevertheless, the conversion is the same. (See diagrams below.)

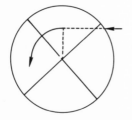 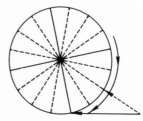

If the point which is about to receive an attack yields slightly, then the external force will slide off and be neutralized. At the instant that the opponent's force is neutralized, the infinite triangles are revolving and each angle is a potential offensive. This is why we say that transforming is striking, or that yielding is striking. Striking is the issuing of energy. Let us ask, then, what is using energy to attack or repel an opponent? (See figures below.)

When issuing energy, it must be directed in a straight line against the opponent's center of gravity. This is like the principle in physics of applying force to a sphere in precise alignment with its center, so that it is prevented from rotating, and it will shoot out like an arrow or bullet. This is the principle of issuing energy in T'ai-chi ch'üan. Whether our energy is directed upwards, horizontally, or downwards all depends upon

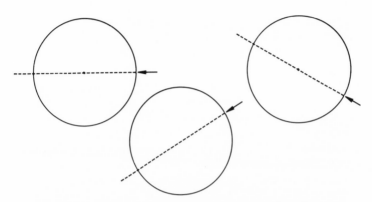

the position of the straight line. One can then issue at will and success is assured. My teacher, Yang Ch'eng-fu, always told me that one should only issue energy after finding the direct line. When issued, it is like shooting an arrow, but this is only for those who have mastered the technique of issuing energy. The principle of the direct line is easily understood, but its application is not certain of success without thorough understanding and experience. Students must concentrate on this point and work conscientiously.

Now someone might say, "I understand the principles you have outlined. However, suppose a man as strong as an ox, as fierce as a tiger, as treacherous as a ram, or as rapacious as a wolf launches a reckless attack which strikes like a bolt of lightning, a veritable thunderstorm bearing down on us with such speed that there is no time to even cover the ears. What shall we do then? I reply that this indeed is a very critical question. What I have already outlined above is precisely the defense against the fierce and rapacious. It is easier than beating opponents who are timid like rats or foxes. The method is complete in what has already been described. With your indulgence, let me set forth these principles once again.

The space occupied by a sphere is greater than any other shape of comparable surface area. Even a surprise attack cannot be more than the sum of two elements: space and time. If the desired speed and effectiveness are not able to control time and space, then the suprise attack is what is colloquially referred to as, "delivering meat to the hook." The outcome is precisely the opposite of his intention, and he has only brought a hasty defeat upon himself. Why is this? A spent bow cannot pierce even a piece of Shantung silk. This is because of the limits of space and also the extension of time, and because of the greater surface and space occupied by the circular form. That is, if we affect the speed by extending the space or time, then there will be a loss of effectiveness. This is the main principle of T'ai-chi ch'üan. I do not resist but yield; I offer no direct resistance but am evasive, causing my opponent's speed and power to be slightly broken. Then following his position I attack, and not even the strength required to blow a hair is wasted. Thus the opponent authors his own destruction within the blink of an eye. This is what the T'ai-chi classics call, "using a pull of four ounces to repel a thousand pounds."[4] This is accomplished precisely by means of what I have just described.

However, this is only one proof, but there is an even higher level. How is an arrow able to fly one hundred paces and pierce seven wooden tablets? First, great strength is exerted to draw the bow and release the arrow. This initial force provides the impetus. The speed of the arrow's motion produces the force of velocity. If we compare the force of velocity with the initial force, they may be equal, or perhaps the velocity is even greater. For example, if the force is one hundred pounds, then the force of the velocity produced may well reach two hundred pounds. If we are able to achieve two hundred pounds, then it is understood that energy is a product of force plus velocity. This may be summarized by the following formula from physics: Force x Velocity x Time = Energy. What is meant in T'ai-chi ch'üan by "using four ounces to repel a thousand pounds" is simply that four ounces of energy is used to turn aside a thousand pounds of power. This is what is meant by force times velocity times time equals energy. When energy has been turned aside and exploited, then of what use is power and speed? Hence, it can be seen that aggressiveness and fierceness alone are unreliable. The power of T'ai-chi ch'üan is thinner than a piece of paper, while the opponent charges us with a force that rushes like the Yangtze and Yellow Rivers. What is our defense? If we confront this force head on, then even a lock a thousand yards long will be of no help. However, if with our single sheet of paper we follow the flow, go with the force and deflect it, then how can the paper be harmed? Now a single sheet of paper may indeed be considered thin, but if employed with speed, it is like attaching it to the shaft of a motor and causing it to spin. When the speed reaches two or three thousand revolutions per minute, then if suddenly the paper should fly off the shaft, it can break even a strong piece of wood. T'ai-chi ch'üan begins with no strength and arrives at great strength. This idea and principle cannot be overlooked. Its function is based on rousing the *ch'i* in the *tan-t'ien* like the waters of the Yangtze and Yellow Rivers, and augmenting this with circular movements. Although the original force is very slight, its speed is limitless. Therefore, its effectiveness is extraordinary and truly immeasurable.

In addition to the function of the isosceles triangle discussed above, offensive postures of the circle and rotating to the left and right or up and down are all based on the function of the lever. T'ai-chi ch'üan takes the fulcrum as the most important part of the lever. The fulcrum is what T'ai-chi ch'üan calls "Central Equilibrium." (See figures below.)

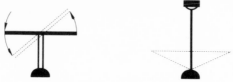

From the diagrams it can be seen that with the exception of the fulcrum, the lever is free to move in any direction, to the left or right, up or down, and back and forth. If, for example, the right side is attacked, then the right side can rotate to the rear.[5] If when one side is about to be attacked, we lengthen the distance and extend the time, then our opponent's aggressive force will be completely dissipated and come to naught. Now, if the force received on the right side of the lever is, for example, one thousand pounds, then the full force of that weight is transferred to the left side. As the right side of the lever rotates rapidly to the rear, the force of the left side rotates rapidly to the fore. Thus the opponent's force has been borrowed to attack him in return, and before he can react, he will be repelled for a great distance. This, then, is the method of issuing energy in T'ai-chi ch'üan. It is as simple as that.

Beyond this, T'ai-chi ch'üan excels at dividing an opponent's strength, as well as using the function of combined forces. (See figures below.)

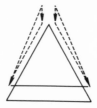 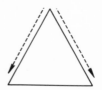

If an opponent presses forward with two hands in a frontal assault, making contact with my two forearms, then I bring them together to form a sharp angle, thus dissipating my opponent's force and reducing it to naught. At the same time, with my forearms together in this position, I borrow the ferocious strength of my opponent to counterattack his vital point. This is what the T'ai-chi ch'üan classics call, "Draw him in and cause his force to fall on nothing. Unite and issue."[6] This is another method.

In addition, T'ai-chi ch'üan also excels at uprooting power, or causing the opponent's root to be pulled up and then throwing him so that both feet leave the ground. This is what the T'ai-chi ch'üan classics call, "If we want to raise something, we must first apply a breaking force, causing the root to be broken, and then we can repel with speed and assurance."[9] This then is the principle of the crane in physics and the lever function of jacks and so forth. (See figures below.)

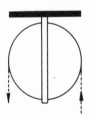

In this diagram, as the distance between the fulcrum and the point of force increases, the force applied decreases and the efficiency becomes greater. In T'ai-chi ch'üan, when employing uprooting energy or issuing energy, we take the opponent as the center of gravity, and the point of contact — hands or wrists — becomes the fulcrum. The feet and legs are the points of force. This is why in T'ai-chi ch'üan, when we issue energy, the point of kinetic energy is in the feet. This is what is called, "The root is in the feet; [energy] issues from the legs, is controlled by the waist, and produces movement in the fingers."[8] Therefore even if the opponent is very strong and imposing, he cannot rely on this, for as soon as contact is made he will be repelled for a great distance. Everything depends on the function of the lever. Although we make contact with the hands, the point from which energy issues is the feet. This is certainly most subtle and supreme. Not only can one expend half the effort and accomplish twice as much, but at its highest, a hundred or a thousandfold. There is absolutely no limit.

To summarize what has been said concerning the movement of energy in T'ai-chi ch'üan and the principles of physics: they are in complete correspondence and are based on the laws of nature. Thus it is apparent that, although T'ai-chi ch'üan's origin is in philosophy, it can be demonstrated by science. In the past, the principles of T'ai-chi ch'üan were so difficult to understand that many people were skeptical. Here by using physics to explain the movement of energy, although T'ai-chi ch'üan is rooted in philosophy, it becomes more easily accessible. Nevertheless, theories of the movement of energy and physics are areas for very deep study in the art of T'ai-chi ch'üan. However, if T'ai-chi ch'üan has its principles, it must also have its applications. If they cannot be applied then the principles are not worthy of discussion. If we seek the perfect unity of theory and practice, then we must thoroughly examine this idea, and only then can we understand the marvelous function of energy in motion. In writing this chapter, the so called secret transmissions of generations of T'ai-chi ch'üan practitioners have been revealed without omission. I hope students will pay special attention to this.

CHAPTER

8

CULTIVATING LIFE
AND MAINTAINING PURITY

"One word can rouse a nation,"[1] and "good government depends on the right man."[2] The state of a nation is simply a function of the talents of its people. Mencius, in speaking of human talent, believed that when great responsibility was about to be entrusted to someone, we must ask what will be their response to hard work and suffering. If one possesses only talent without physical health as a supplement, then what will be the result? Those whose physical health is equal to their talent may be hailed as mighty for a brief time, but when tried and tested by difficulties, before completing a cycle of 60 years, they will already be weak and in decline. If they achieve high office, in their senility they will wrong the common people. What is to be done? As I see it, talent is easy to come by, but true self-cultivation is another matter. Yen Hui[3] died early and Chu Ko-liang was also short lived. Is there any greater loss to the nation than this? Everyone feels sorrow and regret, but no one gets to the bottom of the problem. It is the result of the basket and gourd being often empty as with Yen Hui, or of eating too little and working too much as with Chu-ko Liang and of running about blindly without taking a moment to relax. Mencius said, "I excel at nourishing my great ch'i."[4] This is precisely why Mencius surpassed other men. It is also the reason why Yen Hui and Chu-Ko Liang died early and were not equal to Mencius.

T'ai-chi ch'üan exercise takes cultivating *ch'i* as its primary goal. Sinking the *ch'i* to the *tan-t'ien* may be called, "properly nourishing and not damaging it."[5] Therefore, we follow these words of Mencius. Today, if we wish to emulate Mencius, but are unaware of practicing T'ai-chi ch'üan for the purpose of cultivating *ch'i,* then we must certainly fall short of him. At the same time, to study T'ai-chi ch'üan without understanding what Mencius meant by "abandoning the mind and not knowing how to proceed"[6] I fear will only lead to wearing out one's *ch'i* without benefit. The T'ai-chi ch'üan classics state that the mind and *ch'i* must both be maintained in the *tan-t'ien.* This is "reclaiming one's true mind," "attaining the highest good," "properly nourishing and not damaging the *ch'i,*" and "neither forcing nor forgetting" which causes one's "great *ch'i*" to naturally develop. [7] If one can accomplish this, then establishing the "three imperishables" — merit, virtue, and teachings — is assured of success. In taking up other occupations, one need have no worry. The method is simple and easily practiced. Let me summarize it. Time should never be wasted. We should know which air to avoid and which to take advantage of. Walking, sitting, retiring or reclining, speaking, laughing, eating and drinking all provide an opportunity to cultivate *ch'i.* These three areas are inseparable aspects of our everyday life. Let me discuss them one by one.

While walking or riding, meeting with friends or relatives, listening to lectures or playing chess, we can make use of this time and derive great benefit from maintaining the mind and *ch'i* in the *tan-t'ien.* Sometimes in the morning or evening when the air is fresh and clean, we can concentrate on taking it in. When we smell foul and noxious air, we can hold our breath and turn away. While walking, sitting, retiring, or reclining, we can circulate the *ch'i* in a similar fashion. In the case of walking, however, we must pay attention to distinguishing full and empty in the feet. The foot whose sole sticks to the earth is full; the hand which swings to the rear is also full as *ch'i* flows into the fingers. When sitting, from time to time we should hold an erect posture and straighten the vertebrae of the spine. While standing, one foot should be full, with the sole of the foot sticking to the earth. When fatigue sets in, change feet. When reclining, we should sleep on our right side, with the right leg bent and the back of the left foot against the right leg, just below the knee. The left hand should drape over the left hip, while the right hand cradles the right cheek. The muscles of the whole body should sink and stick to the mattress. In speaking and laughing we should not be too loud, and our *ch'i* should issue from the *tan-t'ien*. If there is saliva, it should be swallowed. We should eat at regular times, and not excessively. We should not hurry, worry, speak or laugh, but sink our *ch'i* as we sit "precariously." The bowl should always be brought to the mouth.

All of this amounts to making the most of our time in order to cultivate *ch'i*. It is simply a matter of "reclaiming our true minds." If we can accomplish this, then there is no time during the day when we are not practicing T'ai-chi ch'üan. This is what I have gained from twenty years of experience. Its benefits cannot be described in words. Even if the basket and gourd are often empty, food is little and affairs are many, why should this bother us? Therefore, I say that in nourishing life, *ch'i* is primary. It is only that those with inconstant minds are not worthy to hear these words.

CHAPTER

9

STRENGTHENING THE INTERNAL ORGANS

The martial arts can be divided into internal and external systems. These are called Shao-lin[1] and Wu-tang.[2] Wu-tang refers to Chang San-feng's internal system of T'ai-chi ch'üan. There is a saying which goes, "The internal trains the *ch'i*; the external trains the muscles, bones, and skin." This indicates the internal system's emphasis on *ch'i*. In *ch'i* training, the ability to sink the *ch'i* to the *tan-t'ien* is of primary importance. When the *ch'i* sinks to the *tan-t'ien,* then it is strong. When the *ch'i* is strong, then the blood is full. When the *ch'i* and blood are strong and full, this is extremely beneficial to the internal organs.

What is the reason for this? The internal organs in man are in some respects different from those of animals. In animals, the spine is horizontal and they are not able to stand erect like man. Nevertheless, although their internal organs are also attached to their spinal column, they are hanging in a series arranged from front to back. With the slightest jump, each organ is able to move backwards and forwards. This enables the main connective tissue attaching each organ to the spine to easily develop strength and fullness. Therefore, this is the reason why animals are stronger than human beings. Because man is able to stand and his spine is erect, the pure and the base can separate, wisdom is sufficient, and he is more intelligent than the animals. It is because of this.

However, the great reduction in man's fierce strength is also due to the same cause. Why? Because the spine is erect, the organs are suspended vertically one on top of the other, piled up and crowded in one mass to the point that the outer membranes of the organs stick to each other. If subjected to the damp heat of summer humidity,³ the spleen and stomach will first be affected. Later, the lungs, intestines, and other organs will suffer disease. No one seems to understand the reason. There is even a belief that if one is a good runner, this will lead to health. In reality, this is very superficial. Being a good runner is certainly better than laziness, but excessive running is injurious to the sinews. Moreover, although the organs are somewhat agitated, they are still piled up and sticking together and cannot enjoy light rubbing contact with each other. In this way, the main connective tissue which hangs directly down, not having the opportunity to move, will surely become weaker and weaker. Only by sinking the *ch'i* to the *tan-t'ien* can this be avoided.

The *tan-t'ien* is located in the abdomen 1.3 inches below the navel. All of the internal organs are above the *tan-t'ien*. When the *ch'i* sinks to the *tan-t'ien,* every time we inhale and exhale, the organs are able to relax and move. With inhalation and exhalation there is opening and closing. When we add movement to this — turning the waist and extending the arms, relaxing the chest and taking steps — then the organs are lightly agitated. Not only does the main connective tissue become daily stronger, but exposure to heat and humidity will not result in illness. Moreover, the strength of our back, heart and brain also increase accordingly. This is a summary of the benefits received. They are the result of sinking the *ch'i* to the *tan-t'ien*, enabling each of the internal organs to be exercised. This then is T'ai-chi ch'üan's benefit to the internal organs. There is nothing else to it. It is not in serving externals, but can only be found internally — only by emphasizing *ch'i*.

CURING TUBERCULOSIS

In my childhood I was weak and sickly. As a young man I served as professor at Y'ü-wen and Yi-shu Universities in Peking. Later I taught in Shanghai at National Chi-nan University and the Shanghai College of Arts. Within ten years I contracted tuberculosis. The cause was inhaling too much chalk dust. Still later I founded the College of Fine Arts in Shanghai.[1] The blackboard there was made of rough glass bricks covered with green felt and erased with a damp cloth. After erasing, it could be used dry or damp. This was specially prepared by colleagues and students in order to avoid following in my unfortunate footsteps. During and after the War of Resistance against Japan, students all across the nation suffered malnutrition. Tuberculosis cases daily increased. I very much pitied them and felt that malnutrition and inhaling chalk dust were major causes in the high incidence of tuberculosis among students. I hope that those involved in education will be concerned with this problem. My own tuberculosis was cured within several months of practicing T'ai-chi ch'üan. However, one case is not sufficient proof. My teacher, Yang Ch'eng-fu, and fellow student Huang Ching-hua, taught this art to countless tuberculosis sufferers who were also cured. Let me briefly discuss, then, its pathology, etiology, and therapy.

Our traditional Chinese medical classics call the lung a "delicate organ." "Delicate" means that it is weak.

However, while recognizing the lung's weakness, they never feared its affliction to the extent of Western medicine. Why is this? Because the lungs are located above the other organs, they are called, "the canopy." They are separate from the digestive system and so cannot be directly reached by injections and drugs. Apart from surgery or rest, they have no idea of any other effective measures. Traditional Chinese medicine emphasizes the "activity of *ch'i*."[2] Especially in cases of tuberculosis, without addressing the "activity of *ch'i*," there can be no successful cure. Therefore, tuberculosis can be more easily cured by Chinese than Western medicine. The history of Western medicine is no more than three centuries. Its progress has been extremely rapid, based on an external approach and proceeding from a study of the material constituents and anatomy of the human body, and aided by sophisticated instruments. As far as the "activity of *ch'i* is concerned, to date they have not the slightest clue. For this reason Chinese and Western medicine have not been able to work together compatibly. This is a great pity!

There are absolutely no effective drugs for tuberculosis. Those who make claims are simply deceiving the public. Why? Direct affliction of the lungs accounts for only three to four per cent of such cases. Besides the lungs themselves, the four other Viscera and Six Bowels[3] can all give rise to lung disorders. Wind, cold, heat, dampness, dryness, and fire[4] as well as the Seven Emotions,[5] Six Desires,[6] and traumatic injuries can all lead to lung disorders. How could one drug cure all of these conditions? What could it be but a fraud? For example, when lung disease results from a stomach disorder, then the root cause is in the stomach. Even if we cure the lung condition, the root will not have been eliminated and the problem will reappear. The same is true of all disorders in the various organs which can give rise to lung disease. Moreover, all of the organs participate in the process of "mutual promotion and inhibition"[9] and if we fail to follow this principle in treating the disease, it will not be successful. Promotion and inhibition is the "activity of *ch'i*." Forgive me for not describing it in greater detail here.

Tuberculosis can only be resisted with spirit and courage; otherwise there will be a rapid deterioration. For example, Ch'en Kuo-fu survived for several decades and was very much himself. When informed of their tuberculosis, those who lack courage become totally dispirited and even relatively mild conditions become more serious. Someone once told me that if his X-ray revealed tuberculosis, he would immediately lie down and never get up. With this attitude, how is a cure possible? There were once two people in my town who became ill. They went to a clinic, and after his examination, the doctor told his nurse that the first man had tuberculosis and should be ordered to rest. The second man, he said, had a cold and should take some medicine. The nurse, however, confused the directions, giving the wrong advice and medicine to the two patients. Before two months had elapsed, the doctor met the first man on the street and noticed that he was in high spirits. The doctor inquired as to his condition, and the man replied that, having been diagnosed as suffering from a cold and taking his medicine, he completely recovered. The doctor was astounded but said nothing. He returned home and sent someone to inquire after the second man, but he had already died. This doctor was a good friend of my fellow student, Ma Meng-jung, and said to him, "Strange indeed is the power of the mind." This was related to me in the spring of 1928.

In the beginning of the winter of 1930, a student, Liu Shen-chan, begged me to cure his brother-in-law,

Mr. Ch'eng, who had been suffering from a severe case of tuberculosis for two years. I agreed. Mr. Ch'eng was the only son of the richest family in Chü-ch'ao. Chinese and Western doctors had all tried in vain to cure him. My student, Liu, told him the following, "My teacher is a remarkable doctor, but he does not lightly consent to cure patients. I approached him with the utmost sincerity and he has agreed to help." He immediately left for Shanghai and came to me for consultation with absolute trust and confidence. After my examination, I lied to him saying that though others had diagnosed him as having tuberculosis, they were mistaken. I told him that despite his fever, cough, and spitting up of blood, with three doses of medicine the bleeding would stop, after which he was to convalesce for ten days and he would be fine. The result was exactly as I said. He remained in Shanghai for a couple of weeks and then went home. A year later I went to Chü-ch'ao and saw him. He was in extraordinary health. So far I have only discussed the role of spirit and courage in cases of tuberculosis, but not yet the disease itself and its cure.

Ignoring for the moment its effect on a patient's spirit and courage, to directly inform a tuberculosis victim of their disease, not only is without any benefit, but can actually hasten their death. When informed of their tuberculosis and ordered to keep to their beds and recuperate, anyone with half a mind will not be able to rest psychologically. Even if they stay in bed and rest, their mental depression might actually be worse than death. In this way, as the body becomes more relaxed, the mind becomes more disturbed. When the mind is disturbed, the "fire" grows hotter and burns the lungs. This is what Chinese medicine calls the "fire of the heart."[8] The lungs belong to the element metal which can be melted by fire. Thus the heart can destroy the lungs and in the blink of an eye burn out of control like a prairie fire. This is unknown to Western medicine. Moreover, to tell a patient that they are in the primary, secondary, or tertiary stage of the illness is tantamount to extending an invitation to death. Is this not a great tragedy?

Tuberculosis sufferers must not spend too much time in bed. When Western doctors see tuberculosis, they invariably advise bed rest. This is a great mistake. The ancients referred metaphorically to the lungs as a "hanging bell." Therefore, when struck it is capable of producing a sound which can carry for a long distance with great clarity. If we rest the bell sideways on the ground and strike it, it will be mute. Thus we can see that it has lost its power. Now, if we make tuberculosis patients lie in bed and not move, the inhalation and exhalation of the lungs cannot freely open and close, and there will be steady deterioration. Under these conditions, how can we expect improvement? Further-more, long periods of reclining causes a reduction in the power of digestion. Even if one's nutrition is good, it will be of no avail. Spending too much time in bed causes a decline in the functioning of the *Tu* meridian. The *Tu* meridian is the spine which is the most impor-tant bone in the human skeleton. When the power of digestion is impaired, the spleen will be weakened.[9] When the functioning of the *Tu* meridian declines, then the kidneys will be harmed. When the kidneys and spleen are both affected, I know of no medicine that can save the patient.

The reliability of X-ray still warrants further study and cannot be considered completely trustworthy. The lungs may suffer from "phlegm-damp"[10] congestion re-sulting in coughing. This may be interpreted on an X-ray as tuberculosis. I have cured many such cases and there is nothing remarkable in this. There are also obstructions caused by "*ch'i* swellings"[11] which can be misdiagnosed in X-ray. When Wu Kuo-chen was head of the Foreign Ministry, his chief of the personnel office was Cheng Chen-yü, an old friend of mine. For a period of some ten years he frequently experienced pain on the left side of his rib cage. He asked me to treat him. I diagnosed his condition as "*ch'i* swellings," but told him that because of the chronic nature of his condition it would take a month to disappear. Because of the length of time required he was not able to undergo treatment. In 1943, while in the United States on official business, his illness recurred. He was examined in one of Washington D.C.'s leading hospitals, and after three series of X-rays was diagnosed as having lung tubercles as large as an inch in diameter. After consultation with noted medical authorities he was told that there was no alternative but surgery. During the operation, an incision was made beginning at the left side of his rib cage and extending to the waist and then the back and diagonally across half the abdomen. In the end no tubercles were found. He very nearly died and received many blood transfusions. Only after six months con-valescence was he able to leave his bed. Chen-yü has many friends who can confirm this. We can imagine then how reliable stethescopes are!

Those in the so called primary stage of tuber-culosis have not yet suffered damage to the *ch'i* or blood, and the disease can be attacked without fear, uprooted, and a favorable prognosis offered. Current methods go no further than this. Tuberculosis patients are not examined from the point of view of cold, heat, deficiency, excess[12] or the influence of ill winds, dry-ness, or dampness.[13] If the patient is immediately given cod liver oil, fritillary and almond extract, vitamins and so forth, this causes the disease to be locked in the lungs and renders it incurable. This is tantamount to cultivating carbuncles or attempting to kill thieves after locking them in. It wastes precious time and is extremely regrettable!

Lung disease is not incurable. I have seen and heard of many cases. Some have recovered by eating large amounts of garlic, or turnips, or millet congee with loquats instead of rice. Others are restored to health by drinking butter.[14] In all of these cases of successful recovery, the approach has been to emphasize attack rather than tonification.[15] I have seen tuberculosis, where there is excessive heat and spitting up of blood, completely cured within two months by eating six raw eggs every morning. Some have also regained their health by eating purslane congee. I have seen people who suffered tuberculosis for many years recover by eating duck force-fed on human placenta. After one night the duck is boiled and eaten for several meals. Some eat boar's lungs prepared by introducing the juice of twelve uncooked baby chicks into the bronchial tubes, stewing in a double-boiler and eating without seasoning. After four or five times some patients get better. I have personally cured many cases of tuberculosis over the past twenty years, even those in the tertiary stage. For Mr. Li Po-t'ing of Sung-chiang, whom both Chinese and Western doctors had given up hope of curing, I prescribed a large dose of cinnamon, aconite root, ginseng, and astraglus root. With one dose there was perceptible effect, with two a lessening of the condition, and full recovery after eight. Later Po-t'ing served as an English instructor at the Whampoa Military Academy.[16] Today, twenty years later, he remains in extraordinary health. In 1932 his youngest son, six years old, developed a fever and stayed in Central Hospital for more than half a year. He was told that it was hereditary tuberculosis. Just at that time I had arrived in Ningpo from Shanghai and prescribed a large dose of cooling medicine,[17] including antelope and rhinoceros horn, foxglove(*rehmannia lutea*) and asparagus root (*lirione graminifolia*). Within a few days his fever abated and he recovered. Today he has already entered college and is in extraordinary health. These are but a few of innumerable examples. As I have already stated, tuberculosis is not an incurable disease. It is critically important to avoid depression, anxiety, and fear.[18] If one can abide by these "three avoidances," then medicine will have a rapid effect. Anger, especially, is most unconducive. Because of my sympathy for the sick, I have tried all methods of curing illness. Therefore, without exhausting all the minor details, I have brought together a number of examples in this chapter for the benefit of those afflicted with illness.

I have said that there is no single specific drug for the cure of tuberculosis and that only T'ai-chi ch'üan is capable of producing unique results. Most people will be skeptical and accuse me of propagandizing or even deception. Let me, therefore, explain more fully. T'ai-chi ch'üan's effectiveness in cases of tuberculosis does not apply to those on their death beds and unable to move, but those who can eat, drink, and walk about. All those who practice will obtain remarkable results. I dare to make this promise regardless of the particular kind of lung disease; all will benefit without the slightest danger. Let me elaborate on some of the main points below.

T'ai-chi ch'üan exercise is what is called "mobilization first and then movement." Mobilization and then movement means that "the mind moves the *ch'i*, and *ch'i* moves the body."[19] Thus we proceed from the inner to the outer, that is from the internal organs to movement of the limbs. This, of course, is based on sinking the *ch'i* to the *tan-t'ien*, which has been discussed in detail in preceding chapters. To summarize again, we emphasize lightness and sensitivity to develop softness, without wasting the slightest energy. We move in such a way as to cultivate *ch'i* and invigorate the blood, relax the sinews and avoid strain. Furthermore, only seven minutes is required in the morning and evening, and it is best not to seek rapid progress.

In sixty to seventy per cent of tuberculosis cases, the cause is exhaustion of the kidneys (gonads).[20] Most often this arises from youthful addiction to masturbation, nocturnal emissions, abnormalities from unsatisfied sexual desires, and incontinence in middle age. In women it often results from irregular periods or a depressed and irritable temperament. From 1940 to 1941 I served as medical consultant for a column in the *Citizens Commercial Daily*. Thousands of readers wrote seeking a cure for their tuberculosis and described the cause of their disease. Thereby I was able to gather much evidence and medical knowledge. The kidneys (gonads) are said to be the "children of the lungs" because the lung's fluids are conveyed to the kidneys (gonads). When the kidneys (gonads) are exhausted, the semen dries up and the lungs are also harmed. As a result, production cannot meet demand. Furthermore, because of deficiency in the kidneys (gonads), the "fire of deficiency"[21] becomes more intense, and the lungs are burned, causing them to dry up. Some become debilitated as a consequence and develop tuberculosis. The lungs are also referred to in Chinese medicine as the "branches" and the kidneys (gonads) as "the root."[22] Just as in the case of a tree, when the root is damaged, the branches and leaves are the first to wither or even fall. How much more so the lungs which are so delicate and weak. There can be no doubt that if the kidneys (gonads) suffer, the lungs will be first to show the symptoms. T'ai-chi ch'üan is a discipline based on sinking the *ch'i* to the *tan-t'ien*, on the complementary interaction of water and fire as in the hexagram "After Completion." Truly this is the one and only method for "strengthening the kidneys (gonads)."[23] When the *ch'i* of the kidneys (gonads) is strengthened, the lungs will gradually recover. This is what I mean by unique results. Who can call it inappropriate?

Deficiency in the spleen[24] can also result in tuberculosis. When the spleen is deficient, the stomach's capacity for absorption will be reduced or the digestion impaired. The spleen is the "mother" of the lungs, thus the lung's *ch'i* relies upon the spleen for sustenance. When there is food in the stomach it must be ground up and transformed by the spleen. When the food is transformed, the *ch'i* is strong. It is first received by the spleen and then transmitted to the lungs. This is why it is considered the mother of the lungs. If, for example, one's belly is starving, the spleen and stomach will first starve, and then the lungs. Faintness of speech or lack of mental acuity both result from the lung's failure to receive nourishment. This is clear. Sinking *ch'i* to the *tan-t'ien* means accumulating *ch'i* in the belly. If deprived of food, one can live for forty-nine days. I once saw this demonstrated by Mr. Su. People say that if food is not taken for seven days, death will result. Some time ago I was staying in Nanking in the home of P'u Chi-p'ing of Chu-p'u and tested this by not eating for eight days. My speech, laughter, and movement remained normal, although my appearance became slightly thinner. This is proof of nourishing the spleen. When *ch'i* sinks to the *tan-t'ien*, the strength of the spleen and absorption of the stomach is increased and the digestion will be good. This strengthens the lungs. We cannot escape the conclusion that this is one of T'ai-chi ch'üan's unique benefits.

When lung disease becomes tubercular and there

is chronic coughing, the lung's *ch'i* is greatly damaged, the body's fluids dry up, and "damp-heat" manifests. As the lungs weaken and become tubercular, then spitting up blood will follow next. It is obvious that when the lungs are weak they have no *ch'i*. By sinking our *ch'i* to the *tan-t'ien*, we accumulate *ch'i*, and the lungs' *ch'i* will be abundant. If this is supplemented by extremely soft, slow, light, and subtle movement, causing the lungs to gradually open and gradually close, then they will never be weak. As long as the lungs are not weakened, the life-force persists, and the processes of elimination and renewal continue. As long as the lungs are not weakened, then even if there is decay, nutrition and medicine will be able to have their effect. As long as the lungs are not totally debilitated, they can gradually come back from weakness to strength and naturally possess the power of rejuvenation. The ability to reverse decay deserves to be called a unique result and is an imperishable truth which I urgently present to those who suffer illness. I have much to say but little space; please forgive my lack of comprehensiveness.

CHAPTER

11

DEFINING THE
STAGES OF DEVELOPMENT

T'ai-chi ch'üan's comprehensive outline is tripar-
tite. The three stages may be designated as heaven,
earth, and man.[1] The stage of man relaxes the sinews
and invigorates the blood. The stage of earth opens
the joints and the stage of heaven involves the function
of awareness. There are nine minor phases with three
in each of the major stages. In the first phase of the
first stage the sinews are relaxed from the shoulders
to the fingers. The second phase is from the groin to
the *yung-ch'üan* point in the center of the ball of the
foot. The third phase is relaxing from the *wei-lü* point
at the coccyx to the *ni-wan* point on the crown of the
head. The first phase of the second stage is sinking the
ch'i to the *tan-t'ien*. In the second phase the *ch'i* reaches
the *yung-ch'üan*. In the third phase it reaches the *ni-
wan*. The first phase of the third stage is listening to
energy. The second phase is interpreting energy. The
third phase is arriving at the level of perfect clarity.
These are the three stages and nine phases. Let me
discuss them in order.

In the first phase the sinews are relaxed from the
shoulder to the wrist. When the sinews are able to
relax, the blood is naturally invigorated. The method
is first to relax the wrists, then the elbows, and finally
the shoulders. Without using any strength we proceed
from total softness. "Seeking always the straight in the
bent,"[2] the form is circular. The bent is unsuitable and

the straight is impermissible. Insufficiencies, hollows or bulges are also impermissible. Finally we will be able to relax the sinews all the way to the tip of the middle finger. This is the first phase of the first stage.

The second phase, from the groin to the heels, proceeds in like manner. The difference is that there are distinctions of light and heavy, empty and full. The foot is capable of supporting the weight of the entire body. This is different from the lightness and facility of hand movements. Most people do not pay attention to full and empty in the feet. Common martial artists also simply follow convenience. Only practitioners of T'ai-chi ch'üan place all of the body weight on one foot, changing feet as required. It is also forbidden to use strength, and we should be relaxed and soft from groin to knees to heels. The power is located in the ball of the foot and is received from the earth. We must distinguish full and empty in the feet and also in the hands. The difference is that if the right foot is full, the left hand will be full. This is the power connection. It is the same with the left foot. The opposite of this is double-weightedness. This is the second phase of the first stage.

The third phase is from the *wei-lü* point to the crown of the head and proceeds in like manner. The spine, composed of many segments, is the most important bone in the human body. From the phrase, "soften the waist so that it can bend in any direction as if boneless," we can see the necessity of softening the spine. This suppleness is made possible by the sinews. The key lies in keeping the *wei-lü* vertical and in imagining that the head is suspended from above. This is the third phase of the first stage.

The first phase of the second stage is sinking the *ch'i* to the *tan-t'ien* and is the foundation for *ch'i* development. The *tan-t'ien* is located in the belly, 1.3

inches below the navel, and nearer the navel than the spine. It is most important that the breath be made fine, long, calm, and slow. Slowly inhale to the *tan-t'ien*, and keeping the mind there as well, hold the breath for a brief moment. After long practice one will experience the ability to suspend the breath.[3] With the passage of days and months, the benefits of "properly nourishing and not damaging" the *ch'i* will be immeasurable. Be completely natural and use absolutely no force. At the outset of study, it is difficult to sink the *ch'i*. If we sink the shoulders and allow the elbows to hang, then the *ch'i* can be guided to the region of the stomach. By slightly hollowing the chest and arching the back, the *ch'i* can sink to the *tan-t'ien*. The opposite of this is when the *ch'i* rises abruptly in an upward direction, resulting in hunched shoulders and elevated lungs. This very easily gives rise to illness. This is the first phase of the second stage.

In the second phase, the *ch'i* reaches the four limbs. After the *ch'i* has sunk to the *tan-t'ien,* it is as if one can direct it with the mind. It is then that we extend it to the groin, the knees, and the heels. This is what is meant by the expression, "the fully realized man breathes from his heels."[4] Then we extend it to the shoulders, elbows, and wrists. When all the joints of the four limbs are open, then it can reach down to the *yung-ch'üan* point in the ball of the foot, up to the *lao-kung* point in the palm of the hand, and terminating at the tip of the middle finger. Thus the T'ai-chi ch'üan classics say, "move the *ch'i* with the mind and the body with the *ch'i*."[5] This is the guiding principle of our practice. This is the second phase of the second stage.

The third phase is the passage from the *wei-lü* point to the *ni-wan*, or what is called, "the opening of the Three Gates," or the first turn of the "inverted movement of the water wheel."[6] However, traversing the *wei-lü* is most difficult; the rest is relatively easy. When one has perfected the practice of sinking the *ch'i* to the *tan-t'ien*, then without even expecting it, the *ch'i* will naturally pass through the *wei-lü*. Absolutely no force should be used or it will result in errors and lead to illness. One must be extremely careful and seek confirmation from trusted teachers. After passing through the *wei-lü*, the *ch'i* rushes through the *chia-chi* point between the shoulder blades, passes through the *yü-chen* point at the occipital bone, and finally reaches the *ni-wan*. This is the threshhold, and one can now make rapid progress towards the *tao*. Longevity and health then follow as a matter of course. This is the third phase of the second stage.

The first phase of the third stage is listening to energy. What do we mean by "energy" and how are we able to "listen" to it? This must be carefully examined. Energy (*chin*) and force (*li*) are very different. Secret transmissions teach that energy issues from the sinews and force from the bones.[7] What marvelous words! Scholars today grope about blindly until the day they die, never understanding the function of energy. This is a great pity! What makes this energy different is simply that *ch'i* which issues from the soft sinews has the quality of flexible power. Only with softness can we stick to and follow our opponent. If we are able to stick, then there is contact between my *ch'i* and that of my opponent. Because we attempt to gauge the movement or stillness of our opponent's *ch'i*, this is called "listening." This, then, is what is meant when the T'ai-chi ch'üan classics say, "When my opponent makes the slightest movement, this is the precise moment for me to move first."[8] This is the first phase of the third stage.

The second phase is interpreting energy. Interpreting energy and listening to energy represent degrees of deep and shallow, fine and gross. I may be able to hear my opponent's slightest movement, but only after being able to interpret it can I move first. Seizing the opportunity and gaining the advantage belongs to me and not to my opponent. This is to progress from shallow to deep. As for fine and gross, this is difficult to describe. The secret transmissions say, "My opponent's slightest movement is heard and known." Slight movements are easily detected, but movement before it manifests is difficult to know. If we can hear and know movement before it manifests, this is very close to the level of perfect clarity. It is simply this; that *ch'i* originates in the sinews, blood vessels, membranes, and diaphragm. Accordingly, we can distinguish four kinds of energy: defensive, hidden, imminent, and parrying. That which shortens the distance between the joints we call sinews. The blood vessels are what circulate the blood. The membranes lie between the muscles and surround the sinews and bones as well as the internal organs. The diaphragm lies above the liver. When *ch'i* issues from the sinews, the situation remains stable and we know that our opponent is on the defensive. When *ch'i* issues from the blood vessels we know that this is the concealment which precedes a change in the situation. When *ch'i* issues from the membranes, we know that it is about to spill over and become manifest, and that our opponent is about to issue energy. When *ch'i* issues from the diaphragm, we know that it is being gathered for a retreat and parry. This is the height of interpreting energy. What could be more subtle or advanced? This is the second phase of the third stage.

The third phase, reaching the level of perfect clarity, is very difficult to describe. One of the T'ai-chi ch'üan classics concludes by saying, "One's mind should be on the spirit and not on the *ch'i*. When it is on the *ch'i* there are blockages. When there is *ch'i* there is no strength. Without *ch'i* there is essential hardness."[9] These words are very strange. They seem to regard the *ch'i* as unimportant. In reality, this is not so. The *ch'i* can be transmuted and evolve into the function of spirit. What is meant by force without force is spiritual force. Wherever the eye focuses, the spirit goes too, and the *ch'i* follows. *Ch'i* is capable of moving the body without the activation of the mind and spirit can carry *ch'i* with it as it moves. This is spiritual force, or what may also be called miraculous speed. In physics, as force is multiplied by speed, its power becomes unlimited. Therefore, spiritual force is the same as miraculous speed. Most scholars overlook the near and pursue the distant,[10] not understanding the marvelous function of the accumulation of *ch'i* in the *tan-t'ien*. *Ch'i* is like wind, water, or clouds, all of which exhibit cumulative force and are one with the accumulated *ch'i* of heaven and earth. This is what Mencius called "cultivating great *ch'i* which at its highest and most substantial fills everything between heaven and earth."[11] This is precisely what I am talking about. The cumulative force of wind and water is easily observed and easily understood. When it comes to the cumulative force of clouds or *ch'i*, it is difficult to observe and to understand. After airplanes came into use, we began to realize that black clouds contained lightening which can utterly destroy absolutely anything it touches. As for the ability of accumulated *ch'i* to support heaven and earth, even less need be said. Spiritual force and miraculous speed contain within them the concept of lightning. This, then, is the evolution of perfect clarity and the third phase of the third stage.

This has been an outline of the stages of development in practicing T'ai-chi ch'üan. Students cannot skip levels, but if they advance by degrees, there should be no difficulty in reaching the highest pinnacle. I emulate the attitude of Chang San-feng and Wang Tsung-yüe [12] and fulfill their unfulfilled ambition. If we abandon this, then methods for strengthening the race and reviving the nation are doomed to superficiality. I hope that students will be diligent.

12

ELUCIDATING
PRODUCTION AND DESTRUCTION

The "Thirteen Postures" include the "eight techniques" and "five steps," which correspond to the eight trigrams and the Five Phases. Ward-off, Roll-back, Press, Push, Pull, Split, Elbow-stroke, and Shoulder-stroke correspond to the eight trigrams: *Ch'ien, K'un, K'an, Li, Hsün, Chen, Ken,* and *Tui.[1]* Advance, Retreat, Gaze-left, Look-right, and Central Equilibrium correspond to the Five Phases: metal, wood, water, fire, and earth. Production and destruction refers to the principle of mutual cyclical production and destruction demonstrated in the theory and practice of martial arts. Metal, in the realm of the martial arts indicates the broadsword. Wood is a staff, water a two-edged sword, fire a spear, and earth a fist. All things are born of the earth. That is, the broadsword, staff, two-edged sword, and spear are all born of the fist.

The use of the broadsword lies in its hardness, and it excels at cleaving. If a staff opposes it, the staff will be split, for metal overcomes wood. The use of the staff lies in its reach, and it excels at thrusting. The term fist refers to the empty hand. If the hand opposes the staff, it will be wounded, and thus wood overcomes earth. Empty hand techniques have the power of grasping. When the sword opposes grasping power, it will be controlled. If the empty hand is able to seize the sword, then earth can overcome water. The use of the sword lies in its softness. When a spear opposes it, the spear will lose its ferocity; thus water overcomes fire. The use of the spear lies in its fierceness, and it excels at piercing. When a broadsword opposes it, the broadsword loses its hardness, and thus fire overcomes metal. This theory has been handed down by martial artists for a long time. Its essence has been outlined above.

However, martial weapons emphasize only mutual destruction, whereas the "five steps" contains the principle of both production and destruction. Take Advance for example. Advance refers to a forward step. Its nature is fierceness, represented by fire. Equilibrium has the power of stability and is represented by earth. When one advances with stability, there is no confusion and victory is assured. Thus fire produces earth. Gazing means gazing to the left. Its nature is hardness and it is represented by metal. We say that if one steps and gazes to the left, then a right fist will follow. If augmented by the power of stability, then earth produces metal. Retreat is the application of softness and is represented by water. Gazing to the left is hard, but if complemented by softness, then metal produces water. Looking refers to looking to the right. Its nature is strong and it is represented by wood. Retreat is soft, but it cannot remain forever soft, so when it is followed by strength, then water produces wood. Advance is fire; its nature is fierceness. With the aid of wood's strength, its usefulness is amplified. Thus wood produces fire. Therefore, it may be said that the "five steps" contain the application of the cyclical production of the Five Phases.

As for the aspect of cyclical destruction in the Five Phases, water overcomes fire, for fire advances with fierceness and water retreats in softness. The hotter the fire, the colder the water. This corresponds to the principle of cyclical destruction in physics. For the rest, refer to my discussion of the sword, staff, and so forth.

The eight trigrams are different.[1] They must be discussed in relation to *yin* and *yang* and the Five Phases, or the principle of what the *I ching* describes as, "[The *ch'i* of Heaven,] the firm and [earth,] the yielding interact, setting the [phenomena represented by the] eight trigrams into reciprocal motion."[2] *Ch'ien*, or Heaven, is metal. *K'un*, or earth, is soil. The trigram *K'an* is water and *Li* is fire. Thus Ward-off, Press, Roll-back, and Push are the four cardinal directions, based on the principle that *yang* is hard and *yin* is soft. This is the fundamental technique of the Thirteen Postures. Although there are four movements, in reality, they are only the application of the two forms — *yin* and *yang*. Among these two, the most strategic is Roll-back. The *I ching* refers to the hexagram *K'an* as "entrapment," calling it doubly dangerous, as the middle lines of the upper and lower trigrams are hard and the outer lines soft. The key to military strategy lies herein. Military strategy is the art of the feint. Military strategists never tire of theories of deception and can never exhaust the marvelous effectiveness of *K'an*, or entrapment and double danger. Therefore, I say that the application of T'ai-chi ch'üan is contained in one technique — Roll-back.

The trigram *Chen*, ☳ thunder, is wood; *Hsün*, ☴ wind, is also wood; *Ken*, ☶ mountain, is earth; *Tui*, ☱ lake, is metal. These are Pull, Split, Elbow-stroke, and Shoulder-stroke, or the four corners of the square. The four sides and four corners combine to form Fu Hsi's arrangement of the eight trigrams, the Primordial Sequence. Pull is *Chen,* thunder, and is *yang*. Its trigram contains both *yin* and *yang*, the image of the ambivalence of full and empty. Therefore, although *Chen* belongs to the element wood, it is also capable of producing fire. This is the basic idea of *Chen*. However, if we want to completely pull up an opponent's rooting energy, then it has the function of testing his full and empty. If the opponent is really full, and I pull him, he will invariably be toppled. If he responds with emptiness, this produces a change in the situation, and I must release him and try another tack. This illustrates the "reciprocal movement of the eight trigrams." If the opponent takes advantage of my Pull and attacks with a Shoulder-stroke, then if I were really pulling, I would be knocked over by his Shoulder-stroke. However, if my Pull is an empty Pull, and my opponent counters with a Shoulder-stroke, he will be striking against nothing. When one strikes against nothing defeat is certain. This is what is meant by, "the firm and the yielding interact," or the fire of *Chen*, wood, overcoming *Tui*'s metal. Split is the trigram *Hsün*, or wind and wood. Elbow-stroke is *Ken*, or mountain and earth. Wood overcomes earth in precisely the same way, so I will not repeat myself. This is because the Five Phases each possess *yin* and *yang*.

Yin and *yang*, empty and full, interact to produce change. This is relatively easy to grasp. However, it is the principle of the changeless within change that is more difficult. The changeless within change is the first principle of the Thirteen Postures. What we mean by change is the alternation of *yin* and *yang*, hard and soft, which produces transformations. Mutual interaction and reciprocity in the Thirteen Postures are all examples of transformation. Changelessness, on the other hand, is the single fixed principle of the essence and function of the Thirteen Postures. This fixed principle is like the stabilizing power of the posture Central Equilibrium. What is the stabilizing power of Central Equilibrium? Central means the "timely response to conditions."[3] Equilibrium is not static equilibrium, but simply not losing our Central Equilibrium. This is the power of stability, or what the *Doctrine of the Mean* calls, "not leaning and not changing."[4] This, then, is the fixed principle of Central Equilibrium.

Changelessness means not worrying about which posture our opponent adopts to attack us. I know that Ward-off and Roll-back are Ward-off and Roll-back. I know that *yin* and *yang*, empty and full are *yin* and *yang*, empty and full. Therefore, I maintain my Central Equilibrium, and am not pulled off balance by my opponent, nor do I pull my opponent off balance. I do not push him, nor do I allow myself to be pushed. This is the fixed principle of changelessness. If I am able to put this into practice, then pulling or pushing are simply mutual transformations. We may execute any technique we like. This is what is meant by, "treading the knife's edge." If one cannot practice the *Doctrine of the Mean,* it is obvious that Central Equilibrium will be difficult. Therefore, I say that the principles and applications of the Thirteen Postures are all based on one posture. The application is called Roll-back, but the principle is Central Equilibrium. There is nothing more to add. "*Yin* and *yang* are called the *tao.*"[5] This is T'ai-chi. It is also the definition of the changeless and the guiding principle of the *Thirteen Chapters.* Is it not fitting?

CHAPTER

13

EXPOSITION OF
THE ORAL TRANSMISSION

As a rule, martial artists who have acquired superior technique keep it secret and do not reveal it to others. It is also customary to transmit it only to sons and not to daughters. However, the sons are not always worthy, and this leads to frequent loss of true transmissions. If, perhaps, a teacher has a favorite student, then he will impart his technique, but always hold something back against unforeseen contingencies. If we go on in this way, can one really expect to see the flowering of our national martial arts?

Although I, Man-ch'ing, studied with Master Yang Ch'eng-fu, I do not dare to claim that I received the full transmission. However, were I to hold things back, or keep secrets and not make them public, this would be to "horde treasure at the expense of the nation."[1] For the past ten years or so, whenever I desired to commit them to paper in order to spread the transmission, this feeling stirred in my mind and I put the task aside. This happened over and over, for I feared the knowledge would reach the wrong people. However, after careful consideration, my sincere desire is to "share the good with others," and so I have faithfully recorded the twelve important oral teachings in order. Master Yang did not lightly transmit these to anyone. Each time he spoke of them, he exhorted us saying, "If I do not mention this, then even if you study for three lifetimes, it will be difficult to learn." If I heard these words once, I heard them a thousand times. To have been so honored by his affection and not been able to live up to his high expectations is a source of infinite shame. Nevertheless, I hope to provide the wise and brave men of the world with the means to study and develop it and enable all people to eliminate illness and enjoy longevity. This would be of profound benefit to the race.

1. **Relaxation.** Every day Master Yang repeated at least ten times: "Relax! Relax! Be calm. Release the whole body." Otherwise he would say, "You're not relaxed! You're not relaxed! Not being relaxed means that you are in a position to receive a beating."

Note. The one word "relax" is the most difficult to achieve. If one can truly be calm, then all the rest comes naturally. Allow me to explain the main idea of Master Yang's oral instructions in order to make them readily comprehensible to students. Relaxation requires the release of all the sinews in the body without the slightest tension. This is what is known as "making the waist so pliant that all of our movements appear boneless." To appear boneless means that there are only sinews. If the sinews are released is there any reason not to be relaxed?

2. **Sinking.** When we are able to completely relax, this is sinking. When the sinews release, then the body which they hold together is able to sink down.

Note. Fundamentally, relaxation and sinking are one and the same. When one sinks, one will not float; floating is an error. If the body is able to sink, this is already very good, but we need to also sink the *ch'i*. Sinking the *ch'i* concentrates the spirit which is enormously helpful.

3. **Distinguishing Full and Empty.** This is what the T'ai-chi ch'üan classics mean by, "The body in its entirety has a full and empty aspect."[2] The right hand is con-

nected in one line of energy with the left foot, and likewise for the left hand and right foot. If the right hand and left foot are full, then the right foot and left hand are empty, and vice versa. This is what is meant by clearly distinguishing full and empty. To summarize: the weight of the body should rest on just one foot. If the weight is divided between two feet, this is double-weightedness. When turning, one must take care to keep the *wei-lü* and *chia-chi* in alignment, in order to avoid losing Central Equilibrium. This is of critical importance.

Note. The word "turning" refers to the pivotal point in the exchange of full and empty. Without revealing this secret, one will never know where to begin. The full energy in the right hand is related to the left hand through a pivot point in the *chia-chi*. The full energy in the left foot is related to the right foot through a pivot point in the *wei-lü*. However, the *wei-lü* and *chia-chi* must be erect and in alignment in order to avoid losing Central Equilibrium. Without sincerely attempting to comprehend these words it will not be easy to accomplish this.

4. Cause the Energy At the Top of the Head To Be Light and Sensitive. This means simply that the energy at the top of the head should be light and sensitive, or the idea of "holding the head as if suspended from above."

Note. Holding the head as if suspended from above may be compared to tying one's braided hair to a rafter. The body is then suspended in mid-air, not touching the ground. In this position it is possible to rotate the entire body, but not to lift or lower the head, or nod it to the left or right. Light and sensitive energy at the top of the head is simply the idea of suspending the head from above. This is all there is to it. When practicing the form, one should cause the *yü-chen* point at the base of the skull to stand out, then the spirit and *ch'i* will effortlessly meet at the top of the head.

5. The Millstone Turns But the Mind Does Not Turn. The turning of the millstone is a metaphor for the turning of the waist. The mind not turning is the Central Equilibrium resulting from sinking one's *ch'i* to the *tan-t'ien*.

Note. "The millstone turns but the mind does not turn" is an oral teaching within a family transmission. It is similar to two expressions in the T'ai-chi classics which compare the waist to an axle or a banner.[3] This is especially noteworthy. After learning this concept, my art made rapid progress.

6. Grasp Sparrow's Tail Is Like Using a Saw. That is, the Roll-back, Ward-off, Press, and Push of push-hands move back and forth like the action of a two-man saw. In using a two-man saw, each man must use an equal amount of strength in order for the back and forth movement to be relaxed and without resistance. If there is the slightest change on either side, then the saw's teeth will become stuck at that point. If my partner causes the saw to bind, then even if I use strength, I shall be unable to draw it back. Only by pushing can I send it back and reestablish the original balance of give and take. This principle has two implications for T'ai-chi ch'üan. The first is to "give up oneself and follow others."[4] By following our opponent's position we can achieve the marvelous effect of "transforming energy" and "yielding energy." The second is, "at the opponent's slightest movement, I move first." That is, when the opponent seeks to push me, I anticipate this by applying pulling force; when he pulls me, I anticipate this by using pushing force.

Note. The metaphor of the two-man saw is really an extremely profound principle. This is a true secret family transmission and one which brought me to a kind of sudden enlightenment. Being adept at anticipating an opponent's slightest movement means that I am always in control and my opponent is always at a disadvantage. The rest goes without saying.

7. I Am Not A Meathook; Why Are You Hanging On Me?

Note. T'ai-chi ch'üan emphasizes relaxation and sensitivity and abhors stiffness and tension. If you hang your meat on meathooks, this is dead meat. How can we begin to discuss sensitive *ch'i*? My teacher detested and forbade this, and so scolded his students by saying that he was not a "meathook." This is an oral teaching in the Yang family transmission. The concept is very profound and should be conscientiously practiced.

8. When Pushed One Does Not Topple, Like the Punching Bag Doll. The whole body is light and sensitive; the root is in the feet. If one has not mastered relaxation and sinking, this is not easily accomplished.

Note. The punching bag doll's center of gravity is located at the very bottom. This is what the T'ai-chi ch'üan classics describe as, "When all the weight is sunk on one side there is freedom of movement; with double-weightedness there is inflexibility."[5] If both feet use strength at the same time, there is no doubt that one will be toppled with the first push. If there is the slightest stiffness or inflexibility, one will likewise be toppled with the first push. In short, the energy of the whole body, one hundred per cent of it, should be sunk on the sole of one foot. The rest of the body should be calm and lighter than swan's down. In this way one can never be toppled.

9. The Ability To Issue Energy. Energy (*chin*) and force (*li*) are not the same. Energy originates in the sinews and force in the bones. Therefore, energy is a property of the soft, the alive, and the flexible. Force, then, is a property of the hard, the dead, and the inflexible. What do we mean by issuing energy? It is just like shooting an arrow.

Note. Shooting an arrow relies on the elasticity of the bow and string. The power of the bow and string derives from their softness, liveliness, and flexibility. Thus the difference between energy and force, the ability to issue or not, is readily apparent. However, this only explains the nature of issuing energy and does not fully detail its function. Allow me to add a few words on the method of issuing energy as often explained by Master Yang. He said that one must always seize the moment and gain the advantage. He also said that from the feet to the legs to the waist should be one unified flow of *ch'i*. He told us that his father, Yang Chien-hou, was fond of reciting these two rules. However, seizing the moment and gaining the advantage are difficult ideas to grasp. I feel that the operation of the two-man saw contains the concept of seizing the moment and gaining the advantage. Before my opponent attempts to advance or retreat, I already anticipate it. This is seizing the moment. When my opponent has already advanced or retreated, but falls under my control, this is gaining the advantage. From this we can see that the ability to unify the feet, legs and waist not only concentrates our power and gives us the ability to "penetrate far,"[6] but prevents the body from being scattered and allows us to hit the mark. The above discussion covers the marvelous effectiveness of issuing energy. Students should study this concept faithfully.

10. In Moving, Our Posture Should Be Balanced, Upright, Uniform, and Even.

Note. These four words — balanced, upright, uniform, and even — are very familiar, but very difficult to implement. Only when balanced and upright can one be comfortable and control all directions. Only when uniform and even can our movement be connected and no gaps appear. This is what the T'ai-chi ch'üan classics mean by, "stand erect and balanced,"[7] "energy is moved like reeling silk,"[8] and so forth. If one does not begin working from these four words, it is not a true art.

11. One Must Execute Techniques Correctly. The "Song of Push-Hands" says, "In Ward-off, Roll-back, Press and Push, one must execute the correct technique." If one's knowledge is not true, then everything will become false. Let me tell you now that if in warding off, one touches the opponent's body, or if in rolling back, one allows one's own body to be touched, these are both errors. When warding off, do not touch the opponent's body; when rolling back, do not allow your own body to be touched. This is the correct technique. During Push and Press, one must reserve energy in order not to lose Central Equilibrium. This is correct.

Note. I had read the words, "One must execute the correct technique," over and over in the "Classic of T'ai-chi ch'üan" without really understanding them. Only after hearing the secret from Master Yang did I realize the proper measure and the correct method. Without oral instruction many things are very difficult to understand. This is often the case. This is an authentic secret teaching in a family transmission. Students should begin with this to experience it for themselves and then they can grasp the proper technique and never lose Central Equilibrium. This is supremely important!

12. Repelling a Thousand Pounds with Four Ounces. No one believes that four ounces can repel a thousand pounds. What is meant by "four ounces can repel a thousand pounds" is that only four ounces of energy need be used to pull a thousand pounds, and then the push is applied. Pulling and repelling are two different things. It is not really that one uses only four ounces to repel a thousand pounds.

Note. By separately explaining the words, "pull" and "repel," we can appreciate their marvelous effectiveness. The method of pulling is like putting a rope through the nose of a thousand pound bull. With a four ounce rope we can pull a thousand pound bull to the left or right as we wish, and he will be unable to escape. But the pull must be applied precisely to the nose. Pulling the horn or leg will not work. Thus if we pull according to the correct method and at the proper point, then a bull can be pulled with only a four ounce rope. Can a thousand pound statue of a horse be pulled with a rotten rope? No! This is because of differences in the behavior of the animate and the inanimate. Man is a sentient being. If someone attempts to attack with a thousand pounds of force from a certain angle, say head-on for example, then with four ounces of energy I pull his hand, and following his line of force, deflect it away. This is what we mean by pulling. After being pulled, our opponent's strength is neutralized, and at that moment I issue energy to repel him. He will invariably be thrown for a great distance. The energy used to pull the opponent need only be four ounces, but the energy used to push must be adjusted to circumstances. If the energy used to pull an opponent is too heavy, he will realize our intentions and find means of escape. An opponent may also borrow our pulling energy, change his direction and use it for an attack. Another possibility is that the opponent, realizing he is being pulled, reserves his energy and does not advance. In reserving his energy, he has already put himself in a position of retreat, and I can then follow his retreat, release my pulling energy and turn to attack. The opponent is invariably toppled by our hand. This is a counter-attack.

All of the above was orally transmitted to me, Cheng Man-ch'ing, by Yang Ch'eng-fu. I do not dare keep this secret, but wish to propagate it more broadly. I sincerely hope that kindred spirits will forge ahead together.

NOTES TO "BIOGRAPHY OF MAN-JAN"

1. Located in Chekiang, Cheng's native province.

2. Located in the southwest part of Szechwan province, Mt. Ch'ing-ch'eng's many caves and beautiful scenery are thought to have attracted the famous Taoist, Chang Tao-ling.

3. *Sun Tzu's Art of War* (*Sun Tzu ping-fa*), China's earliest work on military strategy is first mentioned by Ssu-ma Ch'ien and attributed to Sun Wu of the Spring and Autumn Period. Ye Shih of the Sung was the first to question this attribution and the debate has persisted. Part of the confusion may result from the existence of another Sun Tzu in China's military history, Sun Pin, of the Warring States Period who also authored an *Art of War*. This last work was lost until rediscovered in 1972 during excavation of Han graves in Shantung. There are many foreshadowings of T'ai-chi principles in China's classical writings on military strategy.

4. Chu-ko Liang (181-234) was a prominent figure in the Three Kingdoms Period remembered for his political wisdom and military cunning. Throughout the *Thirteen Chapters* Cheng uses him as a symbol of single-minded devotion to public duty at the expense of personal health.

5. Another statesman and general of the Three Kingdoms Period.

NOTES TO "AUTHOR'S PREFACE"

1. *The Sinew Changing Classic* (*I chin ching*), attributed to Bodhidharma and associated with the "external" or Shao-lin school of martial arts, contains text and illustrations for a series of stretching and strengthening exercises.

2. Vimalakirti, a contemporary of the Buddha, was an enlightened layman, formidable debater, and champion of Buddhist doctrine. Noted for his "skill in means," he manifested disease in his own body in order to attract visitors and preach to them concerning spiritual illness.

NOTES TO "AUTHOR'S PREFACE"

3. *Mencius,* "Kung-sun Ch'ou," Part 1.
4. Yang Ch'eng-fu's *Complete Principles and Applications of T'ai-chi ch'üan (T'ai-chi ch'üan t'i-yung ch'üan-shu).*
5. Festival held on the ninth day of the ninth lunar month, nine being the penultimate *yang* number.

NOTES TO CHAPTER 1

1. *I ching,* "Great Commentary," Book 1, Chapter 11.
2. Approximate quote from *Lao Tzu,* Chapter 36.
3. "Treatise on T'ai-chi ch'üan" attributed by Cheng to Wang Tsung-yüe. (All attributions throughout are according to Cheng and may differ from other editions of the T'ai-chi Classics.)
4. Approximate quote from *Chuang Tzu,* "Yang-sheng chu."
5. *Tso chuan,* Duke Wen, year 18.

NOTES TO CHAPTER 2

1. *I ching,* "Great Commentary," Book 1, Chapter 11.
2. A cursory scanning of the *Nei-ching, Ling-shu, Nan-ching, Shang-han lun,* etc. failed to turn up the term. Until concordances, or at least indexes, to these works become available, we will have to take Cheng's word for this.
3. Collection of nearly 1500 Taoist works. Currently available edition compiled during the Ming, but similar collections were begun as early as the Six Dynasties Period.

NOTES TO CHAPTER 2

4. *I ching*, "Great Commentary," Book I, Chapter 4. Cheng, following orthodox Confucian tradition, considers Confucius the author of this commentary.

5. Also translated as the "Five Elements," metal, wood, water, fire,
   and earth are a fundamental paradigm in Chinese thought used
   to explain cyclical patterns of evolution and correspondences
   between phenomena.

6. Truncated quote from the "Mental Elucidation of the Thirteen
   Postures."

7. Cheng's argument, here, is based on a linguistic device in
   Chinese which is impossible to reproduce in translation. Taking
   the colloquial synonym compound, *"yün-tung"* (exercise, movement), and separately explaining the two characters as "mobilization" and "movement" respectively, he is attempting to bring
   out the special quality of movement in T'ai-chi resulting from
   "sinking the *ch'i*" and Central Equilibrium.

8. The first quote is from "The Treatise on T'ai-chi ch'üan" attributed
   to Wang Tsung-yüe, the second from the "Treatise" attributed to
   Chang San-feng, and the last from the "Song of the Thirteen
   Postures."

9. Truncated quote from "Mental Elucidation of the Thirteen Postures."

10. *Ibid.*

11. *Ibid.*

12. One of the "blockage (*pi*) syndromes" caused by pathogens
    affecting various organs and systems. This one is caused by
    "damp excess" and results in numbness in the limbs and
    localized swelling.

13. Culture hero of the prehistorical Hsia dynasty, who as Emperor
    Shun's minister of water works spent 13 years attempting to
    control the floods, and later succeeded him as Emperor.

14. "Mental Elucidation of the Thirteen Postures."

15. *Ibid.*

16. Allowing *ching*, like *ch'i*, to become a naturalized citizen of the

NOTES TO CHAPTER 2

English language obligates us to a fairly detailed footnote. (The last of the "Three Treasures," *shen*, is adequately, even felicitously in some respects, rendered by the English "spirit.") The colloquial Chinese usage of *ching* often equates simply with the English "semen." However, semen as a translation would be as misleading as giving "breath" for every occurrence of *ch'i*. Current medical definitions of *ching*, based on passages in such classics as the *Su wen* and *Ling shu,* consider it in its pre-natal aspect to be the inherited germ of life and the reproductive potential of the individual, and in its post-natal aspect to be the essential energy derived from "water and grain" which is stored in the internal organs. The seminal essence transmitted from the previous generation is in turn sustained by the extraction of energy from food and so the process comes full circle. Though medical definitions admit also of the two-way transformation of *ching* and *ch'i*, they apply generally to the realm of the normal. To get closer to Cheng's concern in this passage, the super-normal, we must look to the Taoist tradition of inner alchemy. On the Taoist layman's level, one simply attempts to minimize semen (*ching*) loss in order to enjoy health and longevity. In this view, *ching* is compared to lamp oil which is finite rather than well water which is infinite. Other Taoist maxims speak of seven mouthfuls of food being transformed into one drop of blood, seven drops of blood becoming one drop of *ching*, seven drops of *ching* becoming one drop of *ch'i*, and seven drops of *ch'i* becoming one drop of spirit. Untransmuted *ching* will inevitably flow downwards and be lost, but if transformed into *ch'i*, it can be raised to nourish the form and spirit. More esoteric works declare: "*Yin* in the midst of *yang* is *ching*; *yang* in the midst of *yin* is *ch'i*. *Ching* is the mother of *ch'i* and spirit is its child." If the first stage of self-cultivation is simply not taxing the "Three Treasures" in order to establish health, and the second stage (described by Cheng here) is the active (*yu wei*) use of techniques for refining and transforming energy, then the final stage reverts to non-action (*wu wei*) to approach the "formless," the "true," the "primordial," the "pure *yang*," the "fetal," or as Lao Tzu says, "The infant...is innocent of the union of man and

NOTES TO CHAPTER 2

woman, but its penis rises. This is the height of *ching.*"

17. In this context, I believe *"ching-ch'i"* are not coordinate complements, but that *ching* qualifies *ch'i,* so the meaning is *"ch'i* which is derived from *ching.*"

18. "Mental Elucidation of the Thirteen Postures."

19. The idea that *ching* can be refined and used to fortify the brain is a fundamental tenet of Taoist yoga. Various schools split over whether this is best achieved through "paired practices" (*shuang-hsiu, ts'ai-pu* etc.) or solo exercises using the *yin* and *yang* aspects of one's own body. In Chinese medicine, the condition of the bones, marrow, and brain are all dependent on the strength of the kidneys (gonads). In Western terms we might think of this as the conscious sublimation of sexual energy for spiritual work.

NOTES TO CHAPTER 3

1. *Lao Tzu,* Chapter 10. The last two characters, *"chih jou"* (developing softness) were chosen by Yang Ch'eng-fu as the name for his school.

2. *"Ibid.,* Chapter 76.

3. *The Great Learning (Ta hsüeh),* Chapter 1

4. In strictly medical terms, the "heart" (*hsin*) is considered the ruling member of the Five Viscera (*wu-tsang*). It governs blood circulation, but is also associated with many functions assigned in modern Western medicine to the central nervous system and brain.

5. The parameters of the term *shen,* translated here as "kidneys (gonads)," include functions associated with the reproductive, urinary, and endocrine systems and indirectly influences digestion, fluid metabolism, as well as growth and development of the brain, bones, marrow, teeth, hair, saliva, and ears. The gonads

NOTES TO CHAPTER 3

are sometimes called the "external *shen*" *(wai-shen)*, but the *shen* system as a whole is considered the repository of "pre-natal" *ching.*

6. The term "fire *(huo)* has at least three distinct meanings in Chinese medicine: (1) One of the "Six External Pathogens" *(liu-yin,* (2) The heat syndrome of febrile disease, and most relevant here, (3) the *yang* principle or physiological fire of life in various organs, such as the "heart fire," "kidney fire," etc.

7. The heart's charisma is expressed here as the "fire of the ruler." The "fire of the minister" is shared by the liver, gall bladder and Triple Heater, but has its source in the *ming-men* point between the kidneys. The terms "ruler" and "minister" imply distinctions of rank, but also mutual dependence, just as the fifth line in a hexagram is the "position of the ruler" and the second is the "position of the minister."

8. The "Sequence of Former Heaven," or Primordial Sequence, attributed to the mythical Fu Hsi, places the trigram *Ch'ien* (the Creative) at the top (i.e., the South) opposite *K'un* (the Receptive) in the North. King Wen's "Sequence of Later Heaven," however, locates *Li* in the superior position opposite *K'an.* There is a rich tradition in Taoist literature of using the trigrams *Li* and *K'an,* fire and water, to represent alchemical processes.

9. The expressions "substantial fire" *(shih-huo)* and "empty fire" *(hsü-huo)* are generally terms of pathology. In this sense, physiological fire, under the stimulus of internal or external pathogenic factors, may become "fire due to excess" (i.e., *shih-huo)* or, in the absence of sufficient fluid or *yin* principle, may result in "fire due to deficiency (i.e., *hsü-huo).* The distinction here, however, seems to be one of primary versus secondary, real versus delegated power, rather than the conventional medical usage.

10. A point which might be literally translated as the "Gate of Life," but whose location is controversial. Various classical authorities place it in the right kidney, both kidneys, or between the two. It is considered the seat of "pre-natal" *(hsien-t'ien)* or reproductive *ch'i,* and as the locus of "ministerial fire," is sometimes

NOTES TO CHAPTER 3

    called the "lesser heart" (*hsiao-hsin*).

11. See note 9.

12. Collective term for the internal organs. The Five Viscera (*wu-tsang*) include the heart, liver, spleen, lungs, and kidneys. They are considered *yin* because they "store" *ching*. The Six Bowels (*liu-fu*), gall bladder, stomach, small intestine, large intestine, urinary bladder, and Triple Heater are *yang* because their function is to assimilate and transport food. The "organs," it should be remembered, are not anatomical analogues of precise counterparts in modern Western medicine, but rather spheres or systems of function, all with elaborate macrocosmic correspondences and microcosmic relationships.

13. Hexagram 64, "Before Completion" (*wei chi*), features the trigram *Li* (fire) over *K'an* (water). Each following its own natural tendency, rising and sinking, results in a pulling apart or failure of complementary interaction.

14. The stove or crucible is a common metaphor in Taoist yoga for the vessel employed in transmuting bodily substance. Here the *tan-t'ien* (literally "field of the elixir") is the stove, water the "base metal" and mind is the fire. (Cheng does not make the equation explicit here, but water may be taken as *ching* for alchemical purposes.)

15. Hexagram 63, "After Completion" (*chi chi*), is the reverse (*ts'uo kua*) of 64. Here the two trigrams are locked in symbiotic embrace.

16. *Lao Tzu,* Chapter 10.

17. "Mental Elucidation of the Thirteen Postures."

18. The process of achieving "pure *yang*" or immortality is often symbolized in Taoist esoteric literature by the trigrams *K'an* ☵ and *Li* ☲. By borrowing *K'an*'s strong second line, or the primordial fire burning within water, *Li* can transform its weak middle and return to the state of *Ch'ien* ☰, or pure *yang*.

NOTES TO CHAPTER 4

1. The "Six Classics" include: the *Book of Changes,* the *Book of Odes,* the *Book of History,* the *Spring and Autumn Annals,* the *Book of Rites, and the Book of Music* (not extant).
2. *Analects,* Chapter 4, "Li jen."
3. Truncated quote from *Mencius,* "Li Lou," Part 1.
4. That is, they would rather compromise their honor than die as martyrs.

NOTES TO CHAPTER 5

1. From the "Treatise on T'ai-chi ch'üan" attributed to Chang San-·feng.
2. Mythical father of the Chinese race and giver of the arts of civilization. His name coupled with that of Lao Tzu in the compound Huang-Lao is synonymous with the Taoist arts of self-cultivation.
3. Legendary physician of the prehistoric period. The *Classic of Internal Medicine* is framed as a dialogue between the Yellow Emperor and Ch'i Po.
4. *I ching,* "Great Commentary," Book II, Chapter 9.

NOTES TO CHAPTER 6

1. The origins of T'ai-chi ch'üan are the subject of considerable scholarly (and political) controversy. The *locus classicus* for Cheng's assertion is the late Ming (17th cent.) thinker, Huang Tsung-hsi's "Epitaph for Wang Cheng-nan" which states: "The internal stylists (*nei-chia*)...originated with Chang San-feng of the Sung....San-feng was a Taoist of the Wu-tang Mountains." A

NOTES TO CHAPTER 6

"Chang San-feng" is also mentioned in two Ming histories, the Official History of the Ming (*Ming shih*) and Lang Ying's *Ch'i hsiu lei-kao*, but these various accounts are difficult to reconcile. The celebration of his birthday on 1247, the 9th day of the 4th lunar month is based on the biography of Chang in Wu T'u-nan's *T'ai-chi ch'üan* (1928).

2. The term "principle" (*li*) corresponds roughly to our concept of the noumenal, or the realm of natural law collectively called the *tao*. "*Ch'i*" is used here not as elsewhere in the text, but in the sense of the phenomenal or material world. "Image" (*hsiang*) refers to the symbolic significance of what we perceive, particularly the representational value of the lines, trigrams, and hexagrams of the *I ching*. Cheng in the preface to his *Complete I ching (I ch'üan)* calls especial attention to the images as holding the key to the practical application of the hexagrams.

3. The "Eight Extra Channels" (*Ch'i-ching pa-mai*) are those apart from the Twelve Channels and which are not directly connected with the Viscera. The *Jen*, or Anterior Midline Channel, has two branches, the most important of which arises at the perineum, ascends along the stomach, chest, and throat, to the lower lip, where it splits into two lines, ending just below the eyes. The *Jen* Channel connects with and governs all of the *yin* channels. Of the four branches of the *Tu*, or Posterior Midline Channel, the one in question here begins at the perineum and rises straight up the spine to the atlas, where it penetrates the brain, emerging on top of the skull, and descending the frontal bone to the nose, where it terminates at the philtrum on the upper lip. The *Tu* connects with and governs all of the *yang* channels. In his *New Method of Self-Study for T'ai-chi ch'üan (Cheng Tzu t'ai-chi ch'üan tzu-hsiu hsin-fa)* Cheng explains the difference between Shao-lin and T'ai-chi as the former raising external *ch'i* up the *Jen* meridian and the latter raising internal *ch'i* up the *Tu*. (See Wile, trans., *Cheng Man-ching's Advanced T'ai-chi Form Instructions,* p. 13.)

4. *Mencius,* "Kao Tzu," Part 1.

5. Head, arms, and legs.

NOTES TO CHAPTER 6

6. *Mencius,* "Kao Tzu," Part 1.

7. *Ibid.*

8. The "Three Gates" (*san-kuan*) are the *wei-lü* located at the coccyx, the *chia-chi* opposite the solar plexus in the spine, and the *yü-chen* at the occipital bone. The entire circuit connecting the *Jen* and *Tu* meridians is popularly known as the Microcosmic Orbit (*hsiao chou-t'ien*).

9. The first of these quotes refers to the process of transmission of teachings from master to disciple and is derived from Ch'eng I's commentary to the *Doctrine of the Mean (Chung yung)*. The second phrase is from the *Great Learning (Ta hsüeh)*: "Those wishing to cultivate themselves must first rectify the mind." The last is a quote from the *Mencius,* "Kung-sun Ch'ou," Part 1: "At forty I achieved imperturbability."

10. The expression first appears in the *Records of the Grand Historian (Shih chi)* and later in Su Shih's poem "Red Cliff, I" (Ch'ien ch'ih pi fu). In these original contexts the phrase is usually interpreted to mean straightening one's garments and posture and putting on a serious mein.

NOTES TO CHAPTER 7

1. *Moh Tzu*, Book 10, Chapter 40, "Ching shang."

2. "Treatise on T'ai-chi ch'üan" attributed to Wang Tsung-yüe.

3. The trigram *K'an* ☵ pictures one strong line surrounded by two weak lines, *yang* in the midst of *yin*. Among the associations listed for *K'an* in the "Discussion of the Trigrams" (*Shuo kua chuan*), Chapter 10, are "water, ambush, and sorrow." A relevant passage from the text to Hexagram 29 (double *K'an*) refers to the positive applications of entrapment: "The kings and princes make use of danger to protect their realms."

4. "Treatise on T'ai-chi ch'üan" attributed to Wang Tsung-yüe.

NOTES TO CHAPTER 7

5. If translated literally, the text as it stands would read, "For example, if the right side is attacked, the left side can then rotate to the rear." There are basically three reasons for assuming a typographical error here and changing the word "left" to "right." First, if "for every action there is an equal and opposite reaction," then logically, striking the right side should cause the right side to swing away from the impact, i.e., to the rear. Second, Cheng himself a few lines further on repeats his illustration in these words, "Now, if the force *received on the right side* of the lever is, for example, one thousand pounds, then the full force of that weight is transferred to the left side. *As the right side of the lever rotates rapidly to the rear,* the force of the left side rotates rapidly to the fore." (emphasis translator's) Finally, the words *tso* 左 (left) and *yu* 右 (right) in Chinese are easily confused by typesetters, especially when working from handwritten manuscripts.

6. "The Song of Push-Hands"

7. "Treatise on T'ai-chi ch'üan" attributed to Chang San-feng.

8. *Ibid.*

NOTES TO CHAPTER 8

1. *Analects*, Chapter 13, "Tzu Lu."

2. *Doctrine of the Mean*, Chapter 20.

3. Favorite disciple of Confucius who died at the age of 31. The "basket and gourd" mentioned several lines earlier are actually from Confucius' description of Yen, *Analects*, Chapter 6, "Yung ye:" "He had but one basket of food and one gourd to drink."

4. *Mencius*, "Kung-sun Ch'ou," Part 1.

5. *Ibid.*, Also quoted in "Mental Elucidation of the Thirteen Postures."

6. *Ibid.*, "Kao Tzu," Part 1.

NOTES TO CHAPTER 8

7. All of the quotes in this sentence are from *Mencius*, "Kung-sun Ch'ou," Part 1, with the exception of "attaining the highest good" which is from the *Great Learning*.

NOTES TO CHAPTER 9

1. "The Shao-lin Temple in Honan, established in 495, is associated with the birth of Shao-lin boxing and Ch'an Buddhism. Tradition says that Bodhidharma who brought Ch'an (*Dyana*) to China meditated for nine years there facing the wall of a cave.
2. A mountain in Hupeh famous as a retreat for Taoist adepts and the putative birthplace of T'ai-chi ch'üan.
3. A combination of two of the Six External Pathogens (*liu-yin*) described in traditional Chinese medicine as the "damp-heat" syndrome of febrile disease.

NOTES TO CHAPTER 10

1. Cheng taught traditional Chinese painting and calligraphy at all of these institutions.
2. *Ch'i-hua*, literally "process of *ch'i* transformation," is a general term for all physiological processes in the body, including metabolism, catabolism, absorption, elimination, etc.
3. The four other Viscera are the heart, liver, spleen, and kidneys. The Six Bowels are: gall bladder, stomach, small intestine, large intestine, urinary bladder, and Triple Heater.
4. This is the complete list of the so called Six Excesses (*liu-yin*), or abnormal climatic conditions which can have pathogenic influence on the body.

NOTES TO CHAPTER 10

5. The expression "the Seven Emotions and Six Desires" is often used generally to denote the whole gamut of psychological states. Specifically, the term "Seven Emotions" (*ch'i-ch'ing*) is used in medicine to categorize the various internal pathogenic factors, viz., joy, anger, anxiety, worry, grief, and apprehension.

6. The expression "Six Desires" (*liu-yü*) appears in the *Lu shih ch'un-ch'iu*, "Kuei sheng," and there are two Buddhist versions as well. The lists do not match exactly, but generally refer to the senses or sensual gratification.

7. In Chinese medicine the interaction of the Five Viscera is explained according to the Five Phases model. "Promotion" (*sheng*) and "inhibition" (*k'o*) are the normal range of interaction whereby, for example, the kidney's water inhibits the heart's fire, preventing it from overheating, while the liver's wood promotes or fuels the heart. Excessive inhibition results in "invasion," or a role-reversal may produce "insult."

8. The "fire of the heart" is the physiological "fire," or *yang* principle of the heart.

9. In Chinese medicine the spleen (*p'i*) is considered responsible for distributing nutrients, or the "essence of food," to the rest of the body. As such, it is referred to as the "post-natal root." The spleen also plays a role in blood circulation and especially in moving energy and fluids upward to the lungs. Some controversy still exists as to whether the Chinese "*p'i*" refers to the spleen, pancreas, or spleen-pancreas complex.

10. The clinical definition of the "phlegm-damp" syndrome includes large amounts of thin whitish sputum, chest pains, and asthmatic coughing.

11. "*Ch'i-k'uai*," translated literally here as "*ch'i* swellings," seems no longer to be common in current medical usage. Lumps in other parts of the body, such as neck, testes, and skin, are often denoted by compounds consisting of "*ch'i*" plus a specific modifier, and "*ch'i-k'uai*" parallels this construction.

12. These are four of the Eight Diagnostic Principles (*Pa-kang*). "Cold" refers to external invasion by the pathogenic cold factor

NOTES TO CHAPTER 10

or to internal cold due to impairment of the body's *yang*. The same, though opposite is true for "heat." "Deficiency" includes weak *ch'i*, lowered resistance to disease, and impaired physiological function affecting the blood, *ch'i*, *yin*, and *yang*. "Excess" describes rampancy of pathogens and the battle between normal and abnormal within the body. It can also refer to blockages in the body's circulation resulting in excess accumulation and stagnation.

13. These are three of the Six Excesses, or abnormal climatic conditions.

14. The two character combination "*yang-yu*," translated here as butter, is defined in several dictionaries as "kerosene." *Yang-yu* is not the expression in current usage for either butter or kerosene, and the most comprehensive dictionaries such as the *Chung-wen ta tz'u-tien* and *Tz'u-hai* do not list the compound at all. There are two grounds for taking *yang-yu* as butter. The first is the testimony of an informant of Cheng's generation and native province and the second is Robert Dreisback's *Handbook of Poisoning* (ninth ed.) which states: "swallowing causes irritation, vomiting and diarrhea...Ingestion of more than 10 ml may be fatal..." The toxic effects of kerosene actually affect the lungs most severely because of the low surface tension and viscosity of the hydrocarbons which rapidly diffuse into the air sacs during inhalation. It is true that the Chinese pharmocapoeia is broad enough to embrace almost everything under the sun, but if my guess is wrong here, it is only the translation that will suffer.

15. This relates to Cheng's previous statement that tonification or supplementation intended to strengthen the patient's overall health and resistance actually locks the pathogen in the affected organ. Chinese medicine distinguishes three approaches to therapy: "first attack and then tonify," "first tonify and then attack," and "simultaneous attack and tonification." Cheng's recommendation, of course, belongs to the first category.

16. Established in 1924 just outside of Canton City by Sun Yat-sen during the period of Communist-Nationalist cooperation. At one time, Chiang Kai-shek was president and Chou En-lai was chair-

NOTES TO CHAPTER 10

man of the political education bureau.

17. Chinese herbology classifies herbs and their function according to the Four Natures (*ssu-ch'i*) and Five Flavors (*wu-wei*). The Four Natures are cold, cool, hot and warm. Using the law of opposites, Cheng prescribes "cooling" therapy to address heat syndrome symptoms.

18. This is in keeping with the importance given in Chinese medicine to the effect of emotional states on homeostasis, summarized in the Seven Emotions or Five Emotions (*wu-chih*).

19. "Mental Elucidation of the Thirteen Postures."

20. Again it should be emphasized that the term *shen*, often translated simply as "kidneys" includes a number of functions and systems associated in Western medicine with other organs, particularly the reproductive. "Exhaustion of the kidneys" (*shen-k'uei*) is also called Kidney Deficiency (*shen-hsü*). Chinese medicine further distinguishes Yin Deficiency and Yang Deficiency affecting the kidneys. The former is precipitated by excessive loss of semen, while the latter is seen with cold symptoms arising from weakness of the *ming-men* fire.

21. Fire due to deficiency of *yin* fluids.

22. These terms refer to the primary and secondary aspects of the illness. Here the cause is in the kidneys, while the symptoms are most apparent in the lungs.

23. "Strengthening the kidneys" is indicated in Chinese medicine for cases of nocturnal or spontaneous emission, premature ejaculation, or urinary incontinence. The character "*ku*" in the compound "*ku shen*" implies strength in the sense of stability, integrity and resistance to outside influence.

24. "Deficiency," or hypofunction of the spleen may be of two kinds: *yang*-deficiency will manifest as weak spleen function together with cold syndrome, while *yin*-deficiency will present with impaired digestion and absorption along with febrile syndrome.

NOTES TO CHAPTER 11

1. This is a familiar paradigm in Chinese thought and is often called the *san-ts'ai* or Three Levels. The *locus classicus* is the *I ching*, "Great Commentary," Book II, Chapter 10.

2. "Mental Elucidation of the Thirteen Postures."

3. The compound *su-ch'i*, translated here as "suspend the breath," appears also in Chapter 5 of the Thirteen Chapters in his discussion of swimming. As Chinese writings on Taoist yoga use the one word *ch'i* to denote both intrinsic energy and the breath, it is sometimes difficult to untangle the two. Cheng's expression *su ch'i* is not listed in any standard dictionary, and I have not encountered it elsewhere in writings on meditation. Nevertheless, it is clear from context that the meaning relates to the breath and not to internal energy. In Chapter 5 he makes this distinction explicit by using another expression, "*chi ch'i*," when speaking of storing or accumulating intrinsic energy (*ch'i*). In this chapter I believe he is alluding to the phenomena often described in meditation texts as the sensation of temporary breath suspension during states of deep relaxation and absorption. Cessation of the external breath (usually called *chih hsi*) is not a deliberate act, but a side-effect of the gradual lengthening of breath intervals and a shift in focus from the external breath to the inner breath, or what is called the "true *ch'i*" (*chen-ch'i*) or "fetal breath" (*t'ai-hsi*). This is in keeping with the strain in Taoist thought which holds that the key to immortality lies in reducing outflows, including *ching, ch'i,* and *shen.*

4. *Chuang Tzu*, "Ta-tsung shih."

5. "Mental Elucidation of the Thirteen Postures."

6. The compound *he-ch'e* has a number of different meanings in both medicine and meditation, but I believe the operative allusion here is to the water wheel which is capable of harnessing the river's power to move water in the opposite direction of the flow. As such, it is the perfect metaphor for the movement of *ch'i* up the spine or *Tu* meridian during inhalation and down the *Jen* meridian during exhalation.

7. This is discussed at great length in Cheng's *Thirteen Treatises of Man-jan (Man-jan san lun)*. See Wile trans., *Cheng Man-ch'ing's*

NOTES TO CHAPTER 11

Advanced T'ai-chi Form Instructions with Selected Writings on Meditation, the I ching, Meditation, and the Arts, p. 148.

8. "Mental Elucidation of the Thirteen Postures."

9. *Ibid.*

10. This is a common saying so it is not in quotation marks although it does appear in the *"Treatise on T'ai-chi ch'üan"* attributed to Chang San-feng.

11. Slightly truncated quote from *Mencius,* "Kung-sun Ch'ou," Part 1.

12. There are basically two schools of thought regarding the identity of Wang Tsung-yüe. One accepts the Yang family assertion that Chang San-feng created T'ai-chi ch'üan at the end of the Sung and that Wang Tsung-yüe was his chief disciple and transmitter of the art. (See Yang Lu-ch'an's note to the "Treatise on T'ai-chi ch'üan," Yang Ch'eng-fu's preface to *Complete Principles and Applications of T'ai-chi ch'üan,* and Huang Tsung-hsi's "Epitath for Wang Cheng-nan.") The second school, represented by T'ang Hao, Ku Liu-hsin, and Hsü Chen, regard the "Wang Tsung" mentioned in Huang's "Epitath" as not the same person as the Wang Tsung-yüe whom they place in the 18th century and credit with authoring one of the "Treatises on T'ai-chi ch'üan."

NOTES TO CHAPTER 12

1. The Eight Trigrams (*pa-kua*) of the *I ching* constitute the building blocks of the 64 hexagrams. Derived from the doubling of *yin* and *yang* to form the Four Duograms (*ssu-hsiang*), and their doubling, the Eight Trigrams are a basic paradigm in Chinese thought with countless applications.

2. *I ching,* "Great Commentary," Part I, Chapter 1. My translation follows Cheng's own interpretation (See Cheng, *I ch'üan,* pp. 4-5) wherein he expressly differs from Wang Pi. The Legge and Wilhelm translations both follow Wang.

NOTES TO CHAPTER 12

3. The expression "*shih chung*" appears in the *I ching*, Hexagram 4, "Meng" and in the *Doctrine of the Mean*. It is also the name Cheng chose for his school.

4. These words are actually from Ch'eng I's preface to the *Doctrine of the Mean*.

5. *I ching*, "Great Commentary," Part 1, Chapter 5.

NOTES TO CHAPTER 13

1. *Analects*, Chapter 17, "Yang Huo."

2. "Treatise on T'ai-chi ch'üan" attributed to Chang San-feng.

3. "Mental Elucidation of the Thirteen Postures."

4. "Treatise on T'ai-chi ch'üan" attributed to Wang Tsung-yüe. Also *Mencius*, "Kao Tzu," Part 1.

5. "Treatise on T'ai-chi ch'üan" attributed to Chang San-feng.

6. *I ching*, "Great Commentary," Book 1, Chapter 11.

7. "Treatise on T'ai-chi ch'üan" attributed to Wang Tsung-yüe.

8. "Mental Elucidation of the Thirteen Postures."

INDEX

"After Completion," 16, 17, 19

Blood, 12, 46, 52, 54, 55, 57, 60

Bones, 14, 24, 46

Centrifugal force, 32, 33

Centripetal force, 32, 33

Central Equilibrium, 39, 70, 71, 78

Chang San-feng, 8, 27, 66

Chen, 67, 69, 70

Ch'ien, 67, 69

Confucius, 6, 10

Ch'i, 10, 11, 12, 13, 14, 15, 16, 17, 18, 19, 22, 23, 24, 25, 27, 28, 39, 44, 45, 46, 47, 48, 50, 51, 54, 56, 57, 58, 59, 60, 61, 62, 63, 64, 65, 69, 73, 75, 76, 77

Ch'i-hai, ("Sea of Ch'i"), 24

Ching, 13, 14, 15

Ching-ch'i, 14

"Concentrating the *ch'i* and developing softness," 16, 17, 23, 25

Crane, 41

Defense, 34, 37, 39

Doctrine of the Mean, 71

Double-weightedness, 61, 76

Eight techniques, 67

Eight trigrams, 69, 70

Elbow-stroke, 67, 68, 70

Emperor Yü, 12

Energy (*chin*), 63, 76

Fire, 16, 17

Force (*li*), 32, 33, 34, 36, 38, 39, 40, 62, 63, 75, 76

Five steps, 67, 68

Five Phases, 10, 67, 68

Floating, 73

"Four ounces...a thousand pounds," 11, 38, 39

Full and empty, 73, 74

Fu Hsi, 69

Fulcrum, 40, 41

Grasp Sparrow's Tail, 75

Great Ultimate, 8

Hsün, 67, 70
I ching (Book of Changes), 7, 10, 16, 17, 27, 35, 69
Interpreting energy, 8, 60, 63, 64
Investing in loss, 7, 8
Issuing energy, 36, 37, 42
Jen and *Tu* meridians, 27, 28, 53
K'an, 16, 35, 67, 69
Ken, 67, 69,70
K'un, 67, 69
Lao-kung point, 62
Lao Tzu, 7, 16, 17, 18, 19, 22, 24, 27
Lever, 40, 41
Li, 16, 67, 69
"Lightness and sensitivity," 11, 74
Listening to energy, 60, 63
Long Boxing, 23
Mencius, 43,44
Mind, 11, 12, 16, 17, 18, 27, 29, 30, 44, 45, 51, 52, 62, 75
Ming-men point, 17
Moh Tzu, 32
Neutralizing energy, 7, 36
Ni-wan point, 60, 62, 63
Offense, 34
Peking, 49
Press, 67, 69
Pull, 67, 69, 70
Push, 67, 69, 75, 78, 79
Push-hands, 33, 75
Relaxation, 11, 47, 73, 75
Roll-back, 67, 69, 75, 78
Root, 41
Roundness, 31, 33, 34, 36
Saliva, 45
Shanghai, 49, 52, 55
Shao-lin, 46
Shoulder-stroke, 67, 69, 70
Sinews, 19, 24, 47, 60, 61, 63, 64
Sinew Changing Classic, 2
Sinking, 73